THE ULTIMATE GUIDE TO SELF-HEALING

VOLUME 6

LAURA DI FRANCO

Featured Authors: Brigette Burton • Jean Voice Dart • Kelly Daugherty
Dr. Faith Galliano Desai • Johanna Farrimond • Marilyn Fay • Garet Free
Jane Ann Guyette • April Hannah • R Scott Holmes • Sandra Lee
Julianne Thompson Lewis • Melissa T. Maxwell • Laura Mayer
Dr. Tiffany McBride • David D McLeod • DeeAnna Merz Nagel • Donna O'Toole
Rev. Dr. Ahriana Platten • Heather Potvin • Rev. Dr. Karen Schuder
Michele Silva-Dockery • Sensei Timothy Stuetz • Caitilin Twain

25 HOME PRACTICES AND TOOLS FOR PEAK HOLISTIC HEALTH AND WELLNESS

THE ULTIMATE GUIDE TO SELF-HEALING

VOLUME 6

LAURA DI FRANCO

Featured Authors: Brigette Burton • Jean Voice Dart • Kelly Daugherty

Dr. Faith Galliano Desai • Johanna Farrimond • Marilyn Fay • Garet Free

Jane Ann Guyette • April Hannah • R Scott Holmes • Sandra Lee

Julianne Thompson Lewis • Melissa T. Maxwell • Laura Mayer

Dr. Tiffany McBride • David D McLeod • DeeAnna Merz Nagel • Donna O'Toole

Rev. Dr. Ahriana Platten • Heather Potvin • Rev. Dr. Karen Schuder

Michele Silva-Dockery • Sensei Timothy Stuetz • Caitilin Twain

The Ultimate Guide to Self-Healing
25 Home Practices and Tools for Peak Holistic Health and Wellness
©Copyright 2026 Laura Di Franco
Published by Brave Healer Productions
Cover Design: Davide DeAngelis
Interior Design: K.J. Kaschula

Paperback ISBN: 978-1-969999-03-1

eBook ISBN: 978-1-969999-04-8

Dedication

For the Brave Healer community who rallied around me since that morning on March 20, 2020, and said, "Yes, I'll help you write that book!" Thank you for believing in this mission and helping me show the world what's possible! You continue to be the bonfire under this vision.

Table of Contents

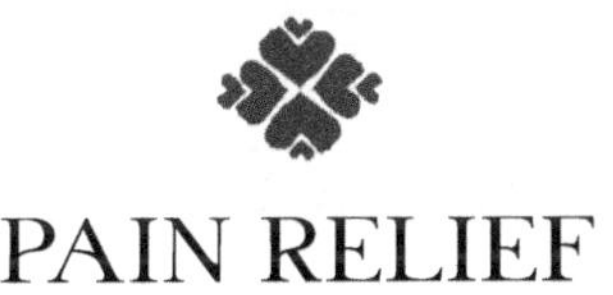

PAIN RELIEF

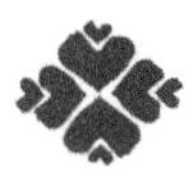

Nervous System Healing

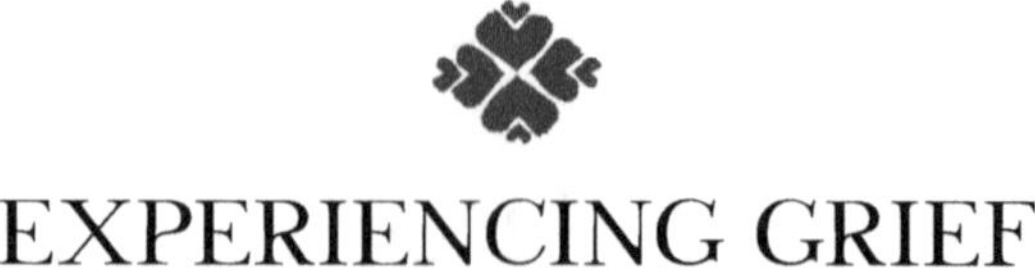

EXPERIENCING GRIEF

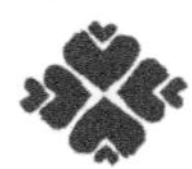

OTHER POSSIBILITIES FOR HEALING

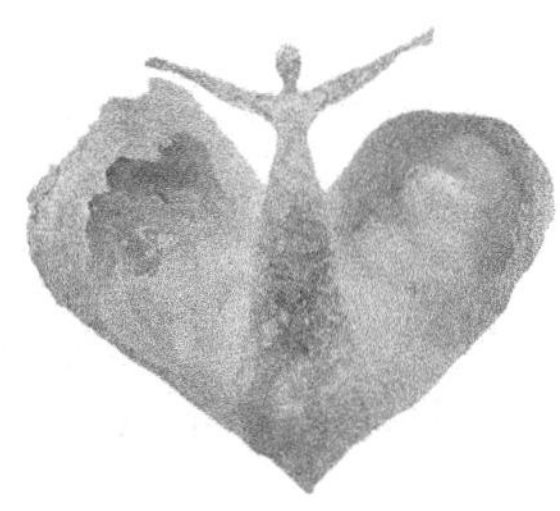

INTRODUCTION

I panicked for about a week after COVID ended my 30-year career as a holistic physical therapist. My identity was fully ingrained in who I was as a healer.

I talked a lot about transitioning before then. "I really want to be full-time with Brave Healer Productions," I said to Mom. But I was too scared to make the leap and risk letting go of the bread and butter. I felt paralyzed.

What if this fails?

Then COVID did it for me; it was the most significant transformation I've ever been through when this tragedy turned into an opportunity.

When I woke on March 20, 2020, I was in a partial dream state when the idea moved through me: *Invite your healer friends to write a book with you. It will be The Ultimate Guide to Self-Healing. The world needs to know how to heal at home right now. It's time to empower people, guide them to their inner wisdom and healer!*

You gotta love that half-dream, half-sleep time in the morning when big messages move through, especially if you're aware enough to hear them.

I got out of bed, walked down the hall to the kitchen in my pajamas, opened up my laptop, and clicked my way to a Facebook group where I taught a business class for holistic healers.

"Who wants to write a chapter for *The Ultimate Guide to Self-Healing?* We'll teach the world all of the self-healing techniques and practices that they can do by themselves at home."

At that point, my community of dedicated holistic health and wellness professionals was growing, and my mission was to help them build their businesses and share their brave words and work with the world in bigger ways. The first class I taught, *Intuitive Writing and Speaking,* marked the beginning of the Brave Healer Productions revolution.

Forty-eight hours after I wrote the note, twenty-four authors said yes. Five weeks later, we had a #1 Amazon bestselling book in multiple categories. That was April 24, 2020. Following the sacred breadcrumbs from the Universe and my intuition (that inner wisdom, voice, and healer) marked the beginning of a world-changing publishing empire.

Whoa, what just happened?

I was excited, but still didn't fully understand the magic the Universe had in store. One week later, one of my friends from the On Purpose Woman community, Lilia Shoshanna Rae, emailed me: "Laura, when are you going to do the next book?"

Well, now I guess!

And here we are, six years later, with *Volume 6* of this world-changing book series.

COVID-19 has literally changed the way this country (and much of the world) works and lives—shutdowns, restricted openings, work-from-home, businesses completely reforming and rewiring the way they do business. With all of this change, the need for self-care and awareness practices has grown exponentially.

In the six years since that morning, Brave Healer Productions has published over 100 Amazon best-selling titles with holistic practitioners and business professionals from more than a dozen countries. Together, we're helping the world experience what's possible. I've never lived my purpose more than now.

When the idea of *The Ultimate Guide* was born, I knew a collaboration was the way to create the most powerful impact. My friend Phil Tavolacci, the author of *What's In Your Web,* got the juices flowing by inviting me to contribute a chapter to his book about the results of John F. Barnes' Myofascial Release. I said yes to three other book collaborations as well. I wasn't a stranger to the idea; I just never saw myself leading one, let alone being a publisher.

After three decades as a holistic physical therapist, one thing I know for sure is that not every modality helps every person, and not every modality helps a person every time they use it. What's most helpful is a toolkit of practices, tools, and modalities to choose from. It's how I practiced as a physical therapist, and it's part of the purpose of this book.

I remember sitting in continuing education classrooms, listening to gurus talk about their modality being *the one,* and that not resonating. I didn't care, though, because my mission was to take the golden nuggets from the class and build my own toolkit. It's what most practitioners do, and it's magic for their clients. As a result, my specialty became complex, chronic pain—that scenario of clients seeing ten different doctors before they get to you. I could effectively handle those clients through my holistic, integrated approach. It's key. Every injury, pain, or illness is a mind-body-soul event. If we don't treat people as the whole picture they are, they won't experience complete relief or sustained healing.

The other thing I knew for sure was that stories heal, both the author and the reader.

The collection of unique, real, and vulnerable stories in these books is one of their biggest gifts. And we need all of the unique stories—every voice—so we can help more people feel hope and connection. Collaborative efforts and energy are world-changing.

These books provide a calm, safe place where healers can tell their whole truth, knowing they're safe and won't be judged. They provide an opportunity to share and realize they're not alone. And readers resonate because our authors' stories are *their* stories. It's healing for the authors *and* our readers.

In May 2025, I marked the milestone of 100 books published with an online event, where the Brave Healer community came together to help me celebrate. It was a moment I'll cherish forever—the realization of the accomplishment, but more than that, the strength of the community that truly cares about the healing journey of mind, body, and soul, and guiding others on that path.

In *Volume 6,* you'll meet 24 of those expert Brave Healer authors who express that same passion to guide, teach, and facilitate this magical process of healing. They're here to empower you to connect with your inner wisdom and healer. **They know that authentic healers don't fix you; they help you connect with the power you have to heal yourself.** In each chapter, you'll enjoy a real story and a practical self-healing tool, as the authors step up as the master teachers they are to guide you in an experience with one of the modalities they love.

With the same spirit and dedication as our original *Volume 1* authors (and all the authors of the volumes in between), we invite you to take a deep breath and explore what's possible for healing. You'll be able to connect with each author to ask questions and continue the journey if you wish.

What if there's something you haven't learned yet that could change everything? It's time to be brave!

With warrior love,

Laura

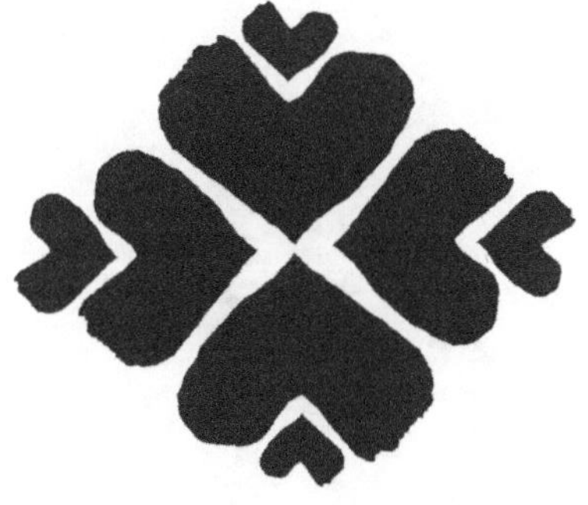

AWARENESS

I chose love in each moment until love was my
new story. I chose gratitude over anger every
moment until gratitude was my new story.
I continue to choose forgiveness and peace over
hatred and regret every moment, and peace is
becoming my new story.

~Laura Di Franco

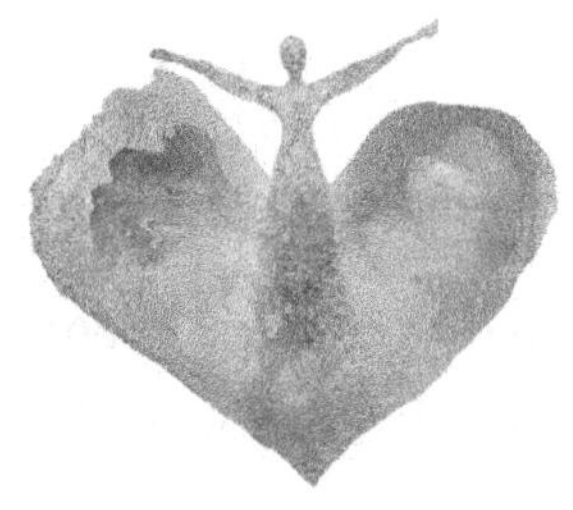

Chapter 1

Brave Story Medicine™
Write Your Way to Peak Performance

Laura Di Franco

MPT, Publisher

My Story

Every word you think, write, or speak creates your current-moment energy and vibration—you're manifesting your life every single moment of every day.

If you're feeling the weight of that, no pressure. This is an opportunity. What else is possible for you right now? What if there's something you haven't learned yet that could change everything?

There came a time recently when I realized: *Shit, I'm responsible for everything in my life.*

And then: *Yes! I'm responsible for everything in my life! This is the ultimate freedom.*

What I can control (my response to life) is the most important thing I can ever control. It's what matters the most. It's the way (through my response of thought and emotion) that I maintain a vibration of love.

Love is the highest vibration next to enlightenment. Knowing I won't be in that highest space constantly, I aim at a practice that brings me back as quickly as possible, especially on the tough days. Writing is my practice; it's my meditation and channel to Divine wisdom. Writing is the way I connect with my higher power. It's also (through intention) how I manifest what I want, including peak health and wellness.

I experienced some pretty crappy life events before these ahas came. I have a list for you to make this as brief as possible:

Death of many loved ones
Death of pets
Divorce
Physical injury (herniated discs in my lumbar spine)
Loss of career
Fighting to send my child's abuser to prison

Some of you have a worse list. I don't think that part matters. We don't win a prize for the most challenging life or the worst tragedy. We're here to live full, juicy, joyful lives. The power is in the choice you have when you're aware: Love or fear.

With awareness, you have a choice.

"You guys, I really don't want to vent about each other's problems anymore. I also don't think we should talk about someone unless they are in the room and can be part of the conversation."

It took courage to share how I want to live with close family and friends. Not venting isn't normal. Most of us complain a lot. We talk about others behind their backs, mostly without ill intent, but still. We focus on problems because it's natural. When I realized I had decades of journals filled with my woes, I had a freakout moment.

Holy shit, look what I've done here! I've spent decades venting, focusing on everything I don't want, and in detail.

I shifted my journaling process last year and also started writing a book called *Write Your Dream Life.*

Every time I write publicly about this, the spiritual bypassing police show up. "You have to feel your feelings," they remind the world. "Don't do that toxic positivity thing."

Y'all, if they really knew me and understood the amount of time I've dedicated to doing the work of healing, the training I've had, the thousands of ours of somato-emotional therapies, and the commitment I made to giving myself permission to feel everything, they'd shut the heck up.

This topic isn't about that. I want you to feel—everything. I want you to get the guidance you need to move through the impossibly painful stuff that's stuck in your mind-body and fascia, and release the trauma. And you can.

What I want you to realize, though, is that through writing (and feeling), you have the power to write your life into reality. Do the work, and then choose something healthier to focus on. Address the pain and grief, and then choose love, joy, and gratitude. Claim those for yourself. Write it down.

Go up to my trauma list and re-read the last entry. As a result of that experience, I've suffered relentless anxiety for going on six years now. This part of my life was not only the most difficult; it also challenged my capacity for stress. I operated on the brink for years. Years! I started telling a story about my life that I ended up repeating (in writing and verbally) for years.

I had another aha last year about this: *This doesn't have to be your story anymore. Who would you be without it?*

So, I started writing a new one about love, healing, forgiveness, and radical abundance. I began living through my writing and Brave Story Medicine™. I chose love in each moment until love was my new story. I chose gratitude over anger every moment until gratitude was my new story. I continue to choose forgiveness and peace over hatred and regret every moment, and peace is becoming my new story.

This is a powerful way to live. It's not easy, because the world will pull you back into bad habits. You're easier to control that way. Some of the healers I know are stuck in those habits, no matter how much they want to believe otherwise. Trailblazing a new story isn't always going to be liked by everyone. That's what makes doing it brave.

***

"The warden at the prison thanked me for coming, Mom. He said victims rarely come to parole hearings. And he told me how much it helps."

"Wow."

I palmed my chest and felt my heart soften a little—my sigh, audible.

"I'm so proud of you. I'm also so glad it's over with for now."

"It was kind of weird. He sat on the other side of a window with his back toward us. He wasn't allowed to turn around."

"Wow!"

OMG, is 'wow' the only thing you have to say?

"Honey, that all seems so weird and stressful. Was it scary going to the prison?"

"I don't know, a little. We had to go through like three locked doors to get inside."

"Sounds like in the movies."

"Yeah."

"I want you to focus on your amazing life, sweet pea. Now that this is done, can you focus on you and healing what you need to heal?"

"I don't know, Mom. I'm going to try."

"Okay. I'm here. I love you so much. You're a very brave, amazing woman. What you did isn't just for you. You fought for every girl who couldn't. Not everyone is as strong or brave as you. When you're ready, try journaling, love bug. Write it all out of you. And then we'll burn it."

"Okay, Mom. I love you."

***

Brave Story Medicine™ is a way to practice body awareness and writing that helps you be aware of and clear old patterns and stories, and choose a new energy and intention for your life. Beyond healing trauma, it's a path to creating the gratitude, love, joy, and health you want to live in every day.

"If you want to clean house, you must first see the dirt." Louise Hay

I write to Feng Shui my soul, first, as a priority for my own healing. But when I took my awareness and journaling practice to another level, it turned into a manifestation tool.

Let's practice.

THE TOOL

BRAVE STORY MEDICINE™
WRITE YOUR WAY TO PEAK PERFORMANCE

You can use writing to heal trauma (a psychology term called narrative therapy), for self-inquiry (to discover your authentic self and purpose), and to manifest your dream life (including peak health and wealth). Your pen is your magic wand. Let's write!

What you need: A quiet, sacred writing space where you won't be distracted and your notebook and pen.

Brave Story Medicine™ has five steps:

1. Journal

2. Read your words aloud to yourself

3. Read your words to someone else/small group

4. Publish your words

5. Speak your words into a microphone

We're going to practice steps 1 and 2 today.

The idea in Step 1 of the Brave Story Medicine™ method is to move words, ideas, thoughts, and beliefs onto the page. If you're worried about someone else reading them, then you can burn the pages later. What's more important is the process because it shifts energy, increases awareness, and heals. If you're worried about hashing up old trauma, think about this for a moment: If the trauma (that is still sitting in your myofascial tissue) is ready to be healed, it will surface. If it's not ready, it won't. You have control here. Be brave.

STEP 1: BE IN YOUR BODY

You can get into any comfortable position and practice any form of body awareness you enjoy. Breathwork and sound healing are my two go-tos. Try noticing what you feel. It's really that simple.

This practice can be more detailed or complex; however, it's really about taking the time to notice what you feel and sense. Do that for five minutes or more. Your body awareness practice is the foundation of using writing to heal and to manifest.

If your mind is full and you have difficulty relaxing, bring your attention to a sound in the room—the air moving through the vents in your home, the buzz of an appliance, the hum of traffic. Allow yourself to sit and relax, just be.

STEP 2: WRITE

After you've cleared your mind and grounded and centered yourself in your body, set a timer for five minutes, grab your notebook and pen, and write as fast as you can without censoring yourself. Fill in the blank:

I feel _____________.

Nowadays, I don't need any prompts, but when I want to use writing as a healing tool and I don't have any ideas to write about, I just use the "I feel" prompt to get me going. There are no rules here. Just write.

When I get stuck (I'm thinking too much and get out of my body), I try to pause for a deep breath or so and start again.

PROMPT #2:

Set your timer for another five minutes and fill in the blank:

What I truly desire for my life right now is ______________.

Write as fast as you can without censoring yourself. Notice the words that want to move onto the page and get out of the way of that process.

NEXT-LEVEL PROMPTS

1. Make a love list. List everything you love so much you lose track of time. Also, list all the ways you love to feel. Practice basking in the feeling in your body with each entry of your list. A love list is an up-leveled version of a gratitude list. Both are nice. Raise your vibe any time by reading your love list.

2. Let's take this to the next level. Once you've cleared some of the thoughts out with the "I feel" and "What I truly desire" prompts and made your love list, it's time to set some focus, energy, and intention on health, wealth, or any other form of peak performance you're interested in creating for yourself.

   Set the timer for another five minutes and write the details of your perfect morning.

   Allow yourself to taste, feel, hear, smell, and see every detail. What does it feel like in your body? Is there anyone there with you? What's that conversation sound like? What do you smell or taste? Write like you're experiencing it now.

   The 'perfect morning' prompt gets you into the energy of the visualized moment, and since your brain doesn't know the difference between that and the actual thing, you'll be "living" that moment now. Have fun with this prompt. Feel and breathe as you write. You're manifesting as you go!

STEP 3: SHARE

This is about adding the vibration of your voice to your words. You can read what you wrote aloud to yourself. You can read it aloud to your friend. Or you can ask your friend to read it to you. Try any version and see what you notice. You may even want to write more about how that made you feel. When you write thoughts down on paper, you create awareness. You become a witness to your own thoughts. When you speak those words aloud, the power of the awareness is amplified. With awareness, you have a choice. You can choose love or fear in those moments. Awareness is life-changing. Writing and speaking are powerful awareness tools.

As someone who shares "out loud" through writing, speaking, and publishing, I'll share a couple more advanced steps for my love warriors. Step 4 (Publishing) is about writing for others to read: blogs, social posts, email newsletters, and books. And Step 5 is about grabbing a microphone. *Eeek!*

I don't do these things without fear, y'all. I just learned how to do them with that feeling inside—how to take action with the feeling. Fear is just a feeling. And it's stealing your show!

In the beginning of my journey, the fight-flight-or-freeze feeling was real—visceral. I shook through being on stage so many times before I got it under control enough to allow me to do it more often. I lost feeling in my legs. I sweat through my shirts.

I've wavered over the last several years, with thoughts like: *Why are you doing this to yourself? Why don't you just live a quiet life and go sell coconuts on a beach somewhere?*

It always comes back to my purpose: to wake the world up to what's possible for healing. We need to be out loud about it. Writing and speaking are the path. Maybe it's yours, too!

To continue being brave and share those words with the world, your purpose has to be burning inside you, not based on what everyone else has taught you what you should want. If nothing else, go back and do that second prompt: What I truly desire for my life right now is__________.

Follow the joy.

Be relentless about that!

Big Warrior Love,

Laura

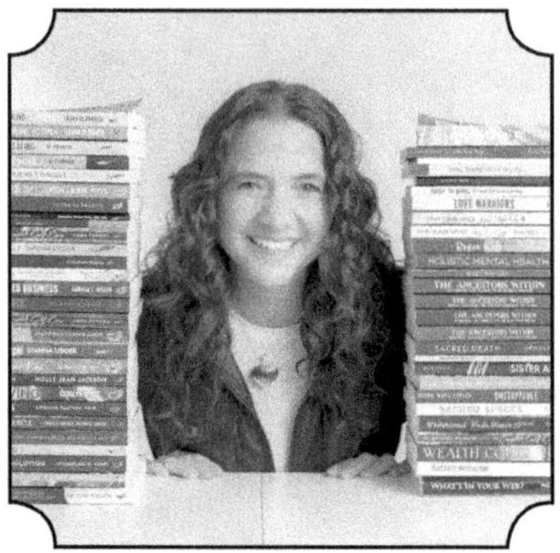

Laura Di Franco is the CEO of Brave Healer Productions, an award-winning publisher for holistic health and wellness professionals and those who serve them. Read more about her in the About the Lead Author section at the end of the book.

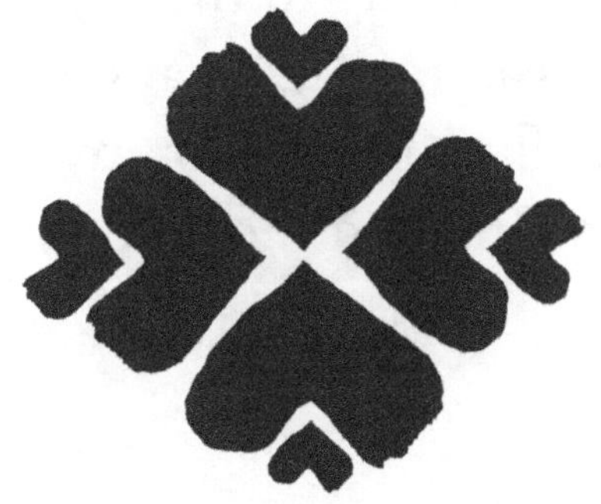

I practiced listening to the language of my body—the tension, fatigue, and gut instincts—until I became fluent. Healing myself became less about knowing and more about noticing.

~ Melissa T. Maxwell

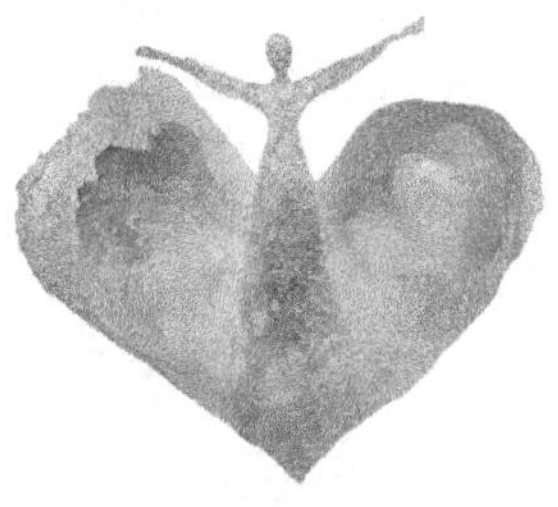

CHAPTER 2

CULTIVATE THE OPPOSITE
YOUR UNIQUE PATH TO RESTORING INNER HARMONY

Melissa T. Maxwell

> ***"Like increases like, and opposites bring balance."***
> ~Ayurvedic principle

MY STORY

"You could die," my gynecologist said, her voice even, matter-of-fact.

She continued despite the startled look on my face. "If your cysts twist, they can cut off the blood supply. It's called ovarian torsion. So, no running, jumping, twisting, or heavy lifting until after surgery."

I could die. I need surgery. This is my nightmare. The room went quiet except for the hum of the fluorescent lights. I stared blankly at the chart on the wall—neat diagrams of organs within my own body that suddenly felt foreign, fragile. My body quietly held this danger, and I didn't even know.

She kept talking—about surgery, risks, medications, next steps—but all I heard was the *ba-dum, ba-dum, ba-dum* of my own heartbeat under the paper gown. The snap of a clipboard brought my focus back to the examination room. I just wanted to get dressed, go home, and think about anything else.

Two months later, in that same room for a post-surgery follow-up, my doctor looked down at her notes, then at me.

"You have endometriosis," she said flatly, almost like I should've known all along. "We'll need to shut your hormones down for a while; put you into medical menopause. It should halt the disease."

I nodded like I understood. But inside, I froze. *Medical menopause? Disease?* My brain catalogued the next steps: research, protocols, nutrition, supplements. If I just figured out why this was happening and what I could do to stop it from happening again, I would be okay. *It was time to get to work.*

For years, working harder was how I avoided what I didn't want to feel—extra classes, taking on every new client, starting a new side business, getting another certification. I loved having a full schedule and feeling busy. Unfortunately, my body had a different opinion and whispered warnings for years, but I just kept silencing it.

The evidence was unmistakable. Painful cramps that knocked me off my feet each month. Fatigue that felt like wading through mud. Erratic mood swings that strained my relationships. "It's normal," I gaslit myself, month after month. *It was not normal.*

"That is a big flippin' needle," I said to the nurse preparing my first injection of the medication for my endometriosis, except I didn't say flippin'. She shook the metallic powder with the opaque liquid in the syringe, creating a mercurial concoction, and turned towards me.

"This might sting, and then your arm may be sore for a couple of days," she warned. I didn't respond, but my face said it all. *Just get it over with.*

The first few weeks of medical menopause were manageable—a few mild hot flashes and some fatigue. I felt cautiously optimistic.

Then, the panic attacks began.

Each episode started as a flutter in my chest, like a trapped bird. Within seconds, my body spiraled—my pulse raced, my chest tightened, my entire body blanketed in heat. "I need some fresh air," I calmly told my husband and friends—not to alarm them—as I sprinted out of the crowded Mexican restaurant, yanking off my sweater, desperate to feel the crisp winter air on my clammy skin. My nervous system felt hijacked, as I spiraled out of control.

Despite the daily panic attacks, I kept coaching and showing up for others. Productivity was my safety blanket. *If I kept moving, maybe I wouldn't have to feel myself unraveling,* I thought. But the more I pushed, the louder my body protested—until every cell seemed to be screaming. *Stop. Listen. Slow down.*

These episodes went on for months, stealing my life. My sleep fractured into restless fragments. My mind, once sharp and steady, turned into incoherent mush. Waves of panic rose without warning, leaving me gasping for air in the most inconvenient places and times.

One particularly rough night, I found myself gripping the edge of my bathroom sink at 2 a.m., drenched in cold sweat. I stared at the stranger in the reflection and groaned, "What the hell is happening to me?" Then, I silently promised myself: *I can't go on like this.*

The next morning, I called my doctor—for the third time in two weeks—to leave another message begging for help or reassurance, but, once again, never received a return call. *I am on my own.*

I started tracking my panic attacks to identify any possible catalysts, and doubled down on what I knew: exercise, clean eating, and supplements. But the harder I tried to control the chaos, the louder it became. My mind was restless, my body exhausted, and somewhere deep inside, I knew, *you can't think your way out of this.*

I lived in imbalance for years—fire feeding fire, movement feeding movement. I tried to fight burnout with gasoline. My body didn't need more intensity and control; it needed the opposite.

The Turning Point

On a warm January evening, about five months into my treatment, I felt the familiar heat and sense of internal suffocation creeping up my body as I sprinted my final lap during a CrossFit workout. My heart raced faster than the clock on the wall, my breath grew labored, and my vision blurred.

The coach saw me pacing with my hands on my head and knew something was wrong. He jogged over to me and asked, "Are you okay?" I barely muttered, "No" between my hiccup-like breaths.

What he did next surprised me. He didn't tell me to suck it up and finish the workout. He just placed a hand on my back and calmly repeated, "You're safe. You're safe. You're safe," over and over, until I almost believed him.

In that moment, I allowed myself to feel safe. I closed my eyes and invited the sensations to roll through me—the heat, trembling, and tears. I didn't try to make them go away or stuff them down. I just felt them.

Surprisingly, something subtle shifted in me. It was a softening—like my body finally exhaled after years of holding its breath and holding everything together. I was cracked open, in a good way. If I wanted to heal, I'd have to learn to listen to and trust my body through the process. *This isn't going to be easy.*

RETURNING TO THE BODY

With a strong background in yoga, I turned to my breath for support. When the panic swelled in my chest, I'd close my eyes and focus on lengthening my exhale, counting slowly to four. Sometimes it worked, sometimes it didn't. Though I noticed when I forced calm, it backfired, and when I softened into the breath, the grip of the hot flash started to release—just a little.

Food became another experiment, but I chose to adjust my approach toward presence rather than control. I paid attention to which foods made me feel grounded versus what triggered my anxiety. Coffee, red wine, raw salads—and other things I once labeled as "healthy"—suddenly felt harsh. I learned to reach for nourishing meals instead—warm soups and stews that made me feel held.

Movement, too, had to change. I used to chase the adrenaline high of intensity, but a brisk walk left me out of breath and overstimulated. I began moving more slowly—gentle stretching and strolls through the woods with my dog. I returned to my yoga practice not for the handstands and chaturangas, but for the savasana at the end.

And then there was my schedule—the invisible weight I'd carried for years. I had to learn to say, "no." No to new clients. No to extra commitments. No to being the dependable one. No to filling every moment with productivity. It felt like failure at first, but over time, the slowing down became medicine, and I began to crave the quiet space between doing. Each no was a yes to my own needs.

As the weeks went on, my body began to trust me again, and vice versa. The hot flashes remained, but the panic softened. I could finally sleep. I could take a deep breath. And through the journey, I uncovered something profound: healing wasn't about controlling my body; it was about changing my relationship to it.

A couple of years later, my studies in Ayurveda, a 5,000-year-old healthcare system from India, gave me the language for what I'd been fumbling towards all along—the principle of *like increases like, and opposites bring balance.* I had lived my whole life on fire—the constant drive, need to control, and the urge to prove my worth—and so my healing demanded the opposite: rest, surrender, and nourishment.

In the end, I didn't find balance in my body through theory. I found it through trial and error, through observing, and through allowing myself to be human. I practiced listening to the language of my body—the tension, the fatigue, the gut instincts—until I became fluent. Healing myself became less about knowing and more about noticing.

I could see how long I'd swept the clues under the rug. Each time I ignored what my body whispered, it spoke louder. The pain, the bloating, the exhaustion—they weren't random. They were the language of everything I hadn't yet let myself feel. Left unattended, those emotions and energies were stored in my body as unmetabolized residue, disrupting digestion, hormone balance, and overall well-being. My symptoms were unprocessed feelings, intensified by medication, asking to be acknowledged.

The following tool is one I return to whenever I feel off-center. It's a simple practice to help you tune in, identify what's present beneath the surface, and gently cultivate the opposite—not to force change, but to remember what harmony feels like.

The Tool

Before you can balance anything, you must first feel it. This is where awareness becomes medicine. When you pause long enough to sense the texture of your inner world, you begin to understand what your body is asking for. Ayurveda offers a timeless language for this awareness, one that helps us make sense of the shifting tides within us.

When you ignore or suppress what you feel, those emotions don't simply disappear; they settle into the body. Unprocessed experiences, stress, or emotions get stored in your tissues, disrupting the natural flow of energy and communication, leading to imbalance. The longer you stay disconnected from what's happening inside, the more those subtle cues grow into symptoms, and ultimately, disease.

Learning to pause and feel what's present is the first step toward release and a way of tending to the body's quiet messages before they turn into screams.

Cultivate the Opposite

Ayurveda teaches us that everything in existence—from the five elements to our sea of emotions—moves according to ten pairs of qualities, or gunas:

1. Heavy/Light

2. Hot/Cold

3. Stable/Mobile

4. Rough/Smooth

5. Dull/Sharp

6. Dense/Liquid

7. Soft/Hard

8. Oily/Dry

9. Gross/Subtle

10. Cloudy/Clear

When one quality becomes overly dominant, imbalance follows. When you invite its opposite, harmony returns. It sounds simple, but the biggest obstacle is noticing what you're feeling in the first place.

Regrettably, we live in a culture that glorifies numbing and overwhelm, rewards analyzing over intuition, and prioritizes fixing over feeling. I'm here to help you rewrite the narrative: self-healing begins with awareness.

This simple tool will guide you to pause, listen, and identify what's true in your body right now, helping you cultivate the opposite of what's depleting you and awaken the intuitive self-healer you've always been.

STEP 1: PAUSE AND FEEL (AWARENESS)

Find a quiet space where you won't be interrupted for a few minutes. Sit or lie down comfortably and close your eyes. Let your breath naturally deepen.

Without trying to change anything, notice what's present in your body.

Ask yourself: *What sensations do I feel in my body—anxiety, numbness, relaxation, warmth, calm, or over-stimulation? Where do I feel these sensations in my body?*

There's no right answer. Your job isn't to diagnose or label, only to notice.

Awareness without judgment shifts your physiology. When you bring gentle attention to what's happening inside—without trying to change or fix it—your body receives the message that it's safe to soften. This kind of awareness invites your nervous system out of defense mode and into a state of regulation, so healing can begin.

STEP 2: IDENTIFY THE QUALITIES (TRANSLATE)

Now that you've tuned in, translate what you're feeling into one or more of the gunas. Your body is always speaking in these qualities, and when you learn its language, you hold the key to your own medicine.

The chart below offers examples of common feelings, their underlying qualities, and the opposite energies that support balance.

Feeling	Dominant Quality	Opposite Quality
Anxious, overthinking	Light, dry, mobile	Grounding, oily, still
Heavy, lethargic, unmotivated	Slow, dense, cool	Light, warm, mobile
Irritable, inflamed, tense	Hot, sharp, intense	Cool, soft, spacious
Numb, disconnected, frozen	Cold, stagnant, dull	Warm, fluid, enlivened
Restless, overstimulated	Mobile, rough, quick	Stable, smooth, slow

You may also notice two or more qualities alive in your body, for example, anxious *and* tense, or heavy *and* cold. That's normal. The body is rarely just one thing. It's always in motion, responding, adapting, and finding its way back to equilibrium.

Sometimes multiple sensations can seem to contradict each other. You might feel both exhausted and wired, or numb yet overstimulated. Instead of judging or labeling them as "good" or "bad," see if you can meet these mixed sensations with curiosity. This is simply your body attempting to self-correct, evidence that it's doing its best to restore balance.

STEP 3: CULTIVATE THE OPPOSITE (ACTION)

Once you've identified the dominant quality, choose one opposite quality to bring in—not as a rigid rule, but as an exploration towards balance.

Ask yourself: *What would the opposite quality feel like in my body right now? What act of self-care brings me this balancing quality?*

Then, choose a small action that supports that new feeling.

Here are a few examples of simple self-care:

If you feel anxious or scattered (light, mobile)

- Wrap yourself in a cozy blanket and take ten slow breaths.
- Eat something warm, moist, and grounding (like vegetable soup or oatmeal).
- Walk barefoot on the Earth or lie on the grass.
- Ground yourself with *abhyanga*—warm oil, full-body massage.

If you feel irritable or overheated (hot, sharp)

- Step outside into fresh air or near a body of water.
- Sip room temperature water infused with mint or rose.
- Try *sitali* or *sitkari* pranayama, a cooling breath practice.
- Take a gentle, unheated yoga class—yin or restorative.

If you feel heavy or stuck (cold, dense)

- Move your body: dance, shake, or go for a brisk walk outside.
- Listen to upbeat music.
- Eat something warm and lightly spiced (like mung bean dal).
- Try a clarifying breath practice—alternate nostril breathing or lion's breath.

Notice that these are small, tangible acts of rebalancing—instead of dramatic overhauls—that you can consistently incorporate until the dominant quality returns to balance. You're not fixing or removing symptoms; you're re-establishing dialogue with your body, guiding yourself to respond rather than react.

STEP 4: REFLECT (INTEGRATION)

After you've invited in the opposite quality, take a few slow breaths and check in again. Journal your answers to these questions:

- What shifted, even slightly?
- How does your body feel now?
- What emotion or sensation has softened or cleared?
- What ritual or practice did you use to cultivate the opposite?

Over time, your notes become a map of your inner rhythm—a record of how you ebb and flow with the seasons, stress, hormone fluctuations, and emotions.

When you look back, you'll uncover patterns:

- Perhaps anxiety peaks when your schedule is over-packed.

- Or you feel heaviness when you've skipped the gym for a few days.

- Maybe your mind feels scattered when you've been mindlessly scrolling on your phone.

- Or your body and mind feel numb when you've repeatedly put off your own needs.

These feelings aren't problems; they're messages from your body, showing you what needs attention so you can respond intentionally (Steps 1-3).

As you continue to practice cultivating the opposite, it becomes less about conscious effort and more about intuitive rhythm. You'll sense imbalance early on—the dryness before burnout, the tension before anger—and have the confidence and clarity to meet it gently with its counterpart.

You'll also learn that balance isn't static. You're not chasing a fixed state of calm or perfection; you're participating in the human experience. Some days will feel fiery, other days will feel dull as ever. The beauty lies in learning how to meet yourself in both.

Each time you pause and feel instead of trying to fix, you surrender a little more to your body's natural intelligence. This is the essence of Ayurveda's ancient wisdom: *like increases like, and opposites bring balance.*

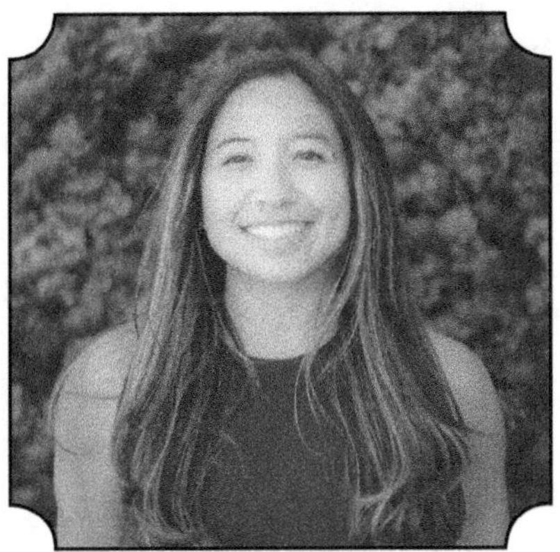

Melissa Maxwell is a certified yoga teacher, holistic health coach, circle facilitator, and writer devoted to helping others become their own best healers by reconnecting with their inner wisdom. With additional training in embodied movement, energy healing, and Ayurveda, Melissa weaves together ancient wisdom lineages with modern, science-backed practices to create multidimensional experiences that nurture whole-person healing.

Her work centers on guiding women and families back to their natural rhythm—living in sync with the seasons and weaving simple rituals into daily life. Through this process of modern rewilding, she helps others tune in to the language of their bodies, nourish their energy, and rebuild nervous system resilience. Melissa believes that true wellness begins when we learn to work with our bodies, not against them.

Melissa's approach is rooted in presence, compassion, and embodiment. Whether teaching yoga, leading women's circles, or writing about the intersection of nature and healing, she invites others to explore what balance feels like in their own bodies. Her offerings are designed to empower others to become their own best healers and to live with more ease, vitality, and connection.

Beyond her professional path, Melissa is a homeschooling mother of two and a lifelong student of life's rhythms. She finds joy in slower mornings, traveling with her family, alchemizing recipes and remedies in the kitchen, and expanding her knowledge—often with a warm matcha latte in hand. She carries a deep curiosity for the world and a gift for fostering connection wherever she goes.

Through her teachings, writing, and community spaces, Melissa cultivates a vision of collective healing—one that bridges the ancient and the modern, the personal and the cosmic, and honors the quiet truth that self-healing begins within.

CONNECT WITH MELISSA:

Links: https://melissatmaxwell.com/links

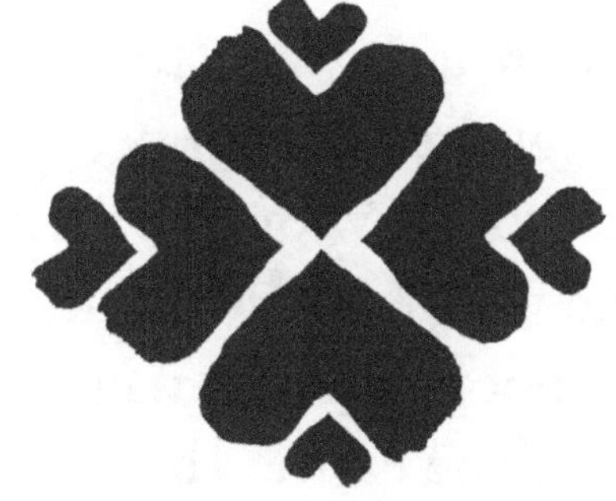

"Long before the word witch was twisted into something to fear, it was a title of reverence. In the old languages of Europe, the root word witan meant to know or to be wise. A witch was someone who knew, who understood the cycles of the moon, the language of the plants, the medicine of the earth. They were the village healer, the midwife of the soul, the shamans who could travel between realms."

~ Dr. Tiffany McBride

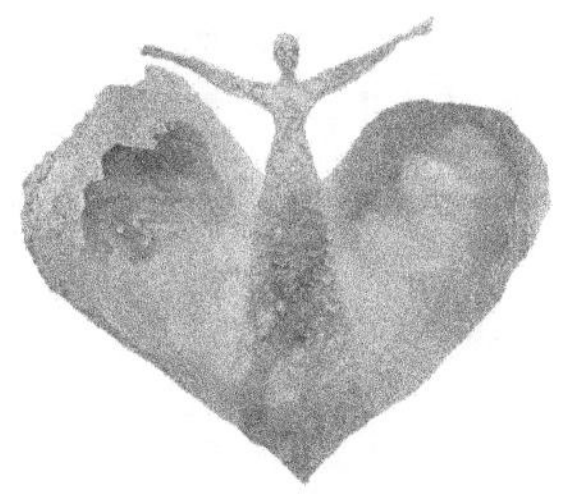

Chapter 3

Are You a Good Witch or a Bad Witch?
Embracing Duality Through the Wisdom of Your Parts

Dr. Tiffany McBride

LCPC, DSPS, RMT, ORDM

My Story

"So are you a bad witch or a good witch?"

People have asked me this for over a decade since coming out as one.

"Of course, I'm a good one!" I say, feeling hurt inside.

Didn't they know who I was?

I once asked someone who flinched at the word *witch,*

"Do you know what a witch is?"

They laughed nervously. "Isn't that, you know. . .someone who worships the devil or does black magic?"

I smiled gently. "That's what we were taught to believe. Do you know where that idea came from?"

They shook their head.

"Long before the word witch was twisted into something to fear, it was a title of reverence," I said. "In the old languages of Europe, the root word witan meant to know or to be wise. A witch was someone who knew, who understood the cycles of the moon, the language of the plants, the medicine of the earth. They were the village healer, the midwife of the soul, the shamans who could travel between realms."

I paused, letting the words settle.

"They weren't evil. They were connected. And that connection, to body, Earth, and spirit, was power."

They tilted their head, eyes softly. "So. . .how did that turn into something bad?"

"When power moves through—through intuition, through the earth itself—it can't be controlled," I replied. "When patriarchal religion rose, it needed intermediaries: priests, institutions, rules. But a witch who could commune directly with the divine in the forest or through her dreams didn't need a gatekeeper. So they were labeled dangerous."

I told them about the sixteenth and seventeenth centuries, when wise women, healers, and herbalists were rebranded as witches, sorcerers, and devil-workers. The Church taught that good spirits could be asked for help but never called upon directly; therefore, anyone who contacted the spirit world was believed to be summoning demons.

"What had once been a sacred relationship," I said, "was redefined as rebellion."

They nodded slowly, eyes wide.

"And that's when the witch hunts started," I said. "Thousands of women, midwives, and healers were tortured and killed. The persecution wasn't really about demons. It was about control: control of knowledge, of healing, of women's bodies and their connection to the other world."

"So a witch was really just a healer?" they asked.

I smiled. "Yes. A wise one. The tragedy is that fear twisted wisdom into wickedness. But the legacy is still alive. Every time we heal through intuition, creativity, and connection to the Earth, we're remembering who we are."

"But aren't there evil witches out there, too? You know, ones that curse and destroy? Someone who uses power for revenge or control?"

"Yes, there are stories for that too," I said. "Do you know the universal story of the two wolves?" I asked.

"Inside of us are two wolves, one is anger, envy, greed, arrogance, resentment, and fear. Sometimes it's referred to as the shadow or the moon. And the other is love, kindness, compassion, humility, and truth, known as the light or the sun. The one who wins is the one we feed."

"Oh yeah, I've heard of that story before," they replied.

"I believe every human has dark and light in them. We all have a wound that we must overcome. My wound in this lifetime was to experience PMDD."

"What's PMDD?" they asked.

"Premenstrual Dysphoric Disorder," I said. "Some people think it's just horrible PMS, but it's not. It's like having Jekyll and Hyde inside of you or being possessed by your own shadow. One part of the month, I'm radiant, social, creative, the sun. Then something shifts, and suddenly I'm the moon—hidden, heavy, pulled by invisible tides I can't control."

They laughed faintly, unsure if I was joking. "So, like mood swings?"

"Not really," I said. "It's not just a mood. It's a full-body takeover. My thoughts shift. My energy changes. It's like the darker wolf takes the wheel and the lighter one gets shoved in the backseat."

They frowned a little. "So what happens exactly?"

"It feels like Hell," I said simply. "Like a fog rolls in over your mind, and nothing makes sense anymore. My chest tightens, my thoughts turn against me, and everything that felt possible suddenly feels pointless. One day, I'm building something beautiful; the next, I'm questioning why I exist at all. It's that sharp, that sudden. I used to think I was broken, or weak, or crazy."

"That sounds hard."

"It is," I nodded. "It's Hell. It used to terrify me. One week I'd feel so alive and creative, like I could take on the world, and then suddenly I'd drop into this pit of rage, sadness, and despair. It wasn't just hormones; it felt ancient, like something deep in my bones. Some months, I'd cry for days. Other months, I'd want to burn everything down just to feel free. There were days I didn't want to live through it; not because I truly wanted to die, but because I couldn't keep cycling through that much pain every single month. Imagine knowing that no matter how good things are, in two weeks, the storm will come again. You start dreading yourself."

They were quiet for a moment. "Did anything help?"

"Not at first. I tried everything: birth control, HRT, supplements, meditation, diets, therapy. Nothing fixed it because no one was looking at the real reason. Years later, I learned I'm neurodivergent, have ADHD, and am autistic. My nervous system doesn't regulate the same way. The hormonal shifts hit me like earthquakes because my brain and body already live at full volume. The world doesn't see how much energy it takes to mask, to hold it all together. So when my hormones drop, the mask shatters. Every suppressed feeling rushes out."

"So what did you do?"

"For a long time, I fought it. I tried to be 'normal.' I tried to control it with anything to silence that dark wolf. But the more I tried to cage her, the louder she howled. She wanted to be seen."

"Seen how?"

"As parts of me that were screaming for my attention," I said quietly. "They were holding everything I hadn't dealt with: anger, grief, exhaustion. The parts of me that were never allowed to exist. Every month, they came back to remind me. To say, 'You can't keep burying this.'"

They sat back. "So PMDD became a kind of messenger?"

"Yes," I said. "Exactly. But I didn't see that at first. I thought it was punishment, something broken inside me. But now I understand—they weren't trying to destroy me. They were trying to get my attention."

"Attention? Parts? What does this all mean?" they asked.

"It means," I said slowly, "that what I used to call my darkness (the rage, the grief, the despair) were actually parts of me. Fragments of my psyche that got frozen in pain, waiting to be heard. In therapy, we refer to it as the Internal Family Systems (IFS) concept—the idea that we're not just one self, but a collection of many selves. Each with its own story, its own wound, its own role."

They nodded, intrigued. "Like inner children?"

"Exactly," I said. "Some parts of me were still carrying things from childhood: rejection, shame, the need to be perfect to stay safe. When my hormones would shift, those parts lost their grip on the mask. They'd rush forward, desperate for care. And because I didn't know how to listen, it came out as chaos."

I took a deep breath. "Carl Jung said something similar: that the goal of life isn't to be perfect, but to become whole. He discussed integrating the shadow, or the disowned and uncomfortable parts of ourselves, and bringing them into conscious awareness. That's what PMDD forced me to do. Every month, I met my own shadow, and every month, she asked the same question: Will you love me yet?"

They were quiet for a moment. "So, the wolves, the parts, the shadow, they're all connected?"

"Yes," I said. "They're different languages for the same truth. Jung called it shadow and light. IFS calls it parts and Self. The old story is called 'The Two Wolves.' But they're all pointing to the same thing, that we're made up of dualities. Love and rage. Joy and sorrow. Creation and destruction. It's not about killing one and saving the other, it's about learning to sit at the table with both."

They smiled faintly. "So everyone has their own wolves?"

"Every single one of us," I said. "Mine just happened to show up through my cycle. But everyone has a dark wolf, a part that holds pain, fear, jealousy, shame, and a light wolf that holds love, creativity, and compassion. The trouble starts when we reject one. When we pretend we're only light, our shadow grows hungry. And when we drown in shadow, we forget the light was ever there."

I looked away for a moment, "The work, the real healing, is to feed them both. To bring compassion to the parts that hurt and awareness to the parts that love. To stop fighting who we are."

"So the goal isn't to make one disappear?"

"No," I said. "The goal is to let them eat from the same hand, to let them know they both belong."

They leaned back, thoughtful. "So before you understood all this, before you found out about the parts, what was life like?"

I exhaled slowly. "Honestly? It was exhausting. I used to work a regular job, and I could never take an actual vacation because I had to use all my time off every month when I didn't feel well. The pain, the fatigue, the depression would wipe me out. I'd use my sick days just to survive, not to rest. It was a continuing cycle. I remember thinking, 'How am I supposed to live like this?'"

They nodded quietly, eyes heavy with empathy.

"So I went out on my own," I continued. "I built a life where I could honor my cycles, where I could work with them instead of against them. I created my own schedule. My own rhythm. My own way of being in the world. Because trying to fit myself into someone else's timeline was destroying me."

"And relationships?" they asked gently.

I gave a small, sad smile. "PMDD ruined a lot of them. I'd swing from love to rage, connection to withdrawal, and I didn't understand why. I thought I was just broken or too much. People called me crazy. I started believing them. The shame was unbearable. But once I began to understand what was actually happening, that my hormones and my parts were reacting, that they were protecting old pain, everything shifted. I could name it. I could communicate my needs. I could say, 'Hey, I'm in the storm right now. I need space, not judgment.'"

They nodded. "That sounds freeing."

"It is," I said warmly. "It's the difference between living at war with myself and living in a relationship with myself. That's what IFS and shadow work have given me: language. Compassion. A map back home."

They looked at me with quiet awe. "So, this isn't just about PMDD."

"No," I said, smiling. "It's about being human. Everyone has their own dark wolf, their own protector parts that rise when life feels unsafe. Mine just wears the face of PMDD. But the lesson is the same; when we listen instead of fighting, we start to heal."

They looked at me curiously. "So are you a good witch or a bad witch?"

I smiled. "Both," I said. "And neither."

"What do you mean?"

"For years, I thought being a good witch meant staying in the light, being kind, loving, calm, and spiritual. I tried so hard to live there that I rejected anything that even hinted at darkness. The anger. The grief. The parts of me that didn't fit the image of 'healer.' But those parts didn't disappear. They just went underground and started casting their own spells; spells of burnout, shame, and self-doubt."

I paused, letting the truth land.

"When PMDD hit, it forced me to face that shadow. Every month, I met the bad witch inside me, the one who wanted to scream, destroy, burn it all down. For a long time, I was terrified of her. But eventually, I realized she wasn't evil. She was the keeper of my power, the side that refused to be silenced. She was the voice saying, Something is not right. Something in you needs to be seen."

"So the bad witch was really. . .trying to help?"

"Exactly," I said. "She was protecting me the only way she knew how. Once I started listening to her, to my parts, my dark wolf, everything began to shift. I didn't have to destroy her to be good. I just had to love her, too."

I leaned in a little, my tone gentle. "The truth is, we're all witches. Every single one of us. We all work with energy—our words, our choices, our emotions, casting spells with how we show up in the world. Some of us feed the dark witch: resentment, fear, control. Some feed only the light witch: positivity, denial, avoidance. But real magic, real healing, comes when we learn to feed them both. To love them both. To let them work together."

They were quiet for a long time. "So it's not really about being good or bad," they said.

"No," I whispered. "It's about being whole."

The Tool

Duality is one of life's oldest teachers.

It exists in every sunrise and sunset, in the inhale and the exhale, in birth and death, in stillness and motion. Within each of us lives this same rhythm: the light and the shadow, the healer and the wounded one, the witch who blesses and the witch who burns.

We are taught to pick one side—to be good, kind, calm, spiritual, productive—and to hide the rest. But wholeness isn't about choosing sides; it's about learning to hold them both.

In Jungian terminology, this refers to the integration of the shadow and the light.

In Internal Family Systems, it's befriending your parts.

In the old stories, it's feeding both wolves.

These are all different ways of saying the same truth:

You are not broken.

You are multifaceted.

You are a constellation of selves, each one trying to help you survive, to protect you, to love you in the only way it knows how.

Some parts carry pain: the protector, the controller, the angry one, the avoider.

Some parts carry purity: the lover, the dreamer, the healer, the creator.

Each is shaped by your experiences, your nervous system, and your ancestry.

Each holds wisdom.

When you reject or exile a part, it doesn't disappear; it becomes louder. It attempts to capture your attention through the body, emotions, illness, or exhaustion. That's what my darkest seasons did through PMDD. Each month, they came back to say, 'There's something you're not listening to.' The rage, grief, and hopelessness, they weren't trying to destroy me. They were trying to speak for the parts of me that had been silenced.

That's the work of shadow integration, to turn toward the parts we fear, to listen without judgment, and to see the sacred intention behind the chaos.

SOMATIC PARTS CHECK-IN

Find a quiet, comfortable place. Allow yourself to be supported—your body on the chair, the ground, or the bed beneath you.

1. Arrive in the body.

   Take a slow breath in through your nose and exhale through your mouth.

   Notice the natural rhythm of your breathing.

   Feel where your body meets the surface beneath you.

   Let your shoulders soften, your jaw unclench, your belly expand.

2. Sense.

   Bring your attention inside.

   Without needing to change anything, notice what's present in your body right now: pressure, tightness, warmth, tingling, numbness, stillness.

Simply name what you feel: *There is heaviness in my chest. There is fluttering in my stomach.*

Each sensation is a messenger, a doorway to a part of you.

3. Invite curiosity.

   Ask quietly inside:

   Is there a part of me that wants my attention right now?

   Wait. See what arises—maybe a feeling, image, memory, or simply a sense of presence.

   If something comes forward, breathe gently and ask:

   - *How long have you been here?*
   - *What are you trying to help me with?*
   - *What do you need me to be aware of?*

   There are no correct answers. Listen with the same patience you would offer a dear friend.

4. Acknowledge.

   When a part shares something—a fear, story, sensation—thank it for showing up.

   You might say silently or aloud:

   "Thank you for protecting me."

   "I see how hard you've been working."

   "You don't have to do this alone anymore."

   Notice any slight shifts—a deeper breath, warmth, or relaxation.

   That's the body signaling safety.

5. Expand awareness.

    Now, bring your attention to the rest of your system.

    Are there other parts nearby that feel calm, creative, and compassionate?

    These supportive energies are also you.

    Let them hold space for the parts that are tired or afraid.

6. Integrate.

    Take a few breaths, sensing all of yourself at once—the sensations, emotions, thoughts, and awareness that coexist within you.

    This is duality in motion: your inner world learning to be together—not in conflict, but in conversation.

7. Close gently.

    Place a hand over your heart.

    Feel the steady rhythm beneath your palm.

    Whisper, if it feels right:

    "All of me is welcome here."

    Stay for a moment in the truth that nothing inside you needs to be exiled for you to be whole.

    When you're ready, slowly open your eyes, noticing the light, the sounds, and the ground beneath you.

    If you'd like to deepen this practice, you can listen to my guided somatic parts meditation—a gentle recording that guides you through this process with breath, music, and embodied awareness.

    Find it at https://www.tiffany-mcbride.org/meditations.

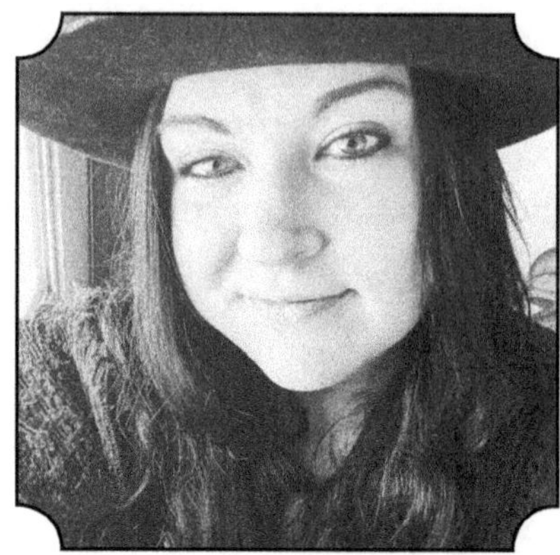

Dr. Tiffany McBride is a Doctor of Shamanic Psycho-Spiritual Studies, a Healing Arts Minister, and a Creative Coach, devoted to the alchemy of healing, artistry, and soul embodiment. A clinical psychotherapist turned mystic, she bridges the worlds of science and spirit, shadow and light, trauma and transformation.

With over two decades of experience, Tiffany holds advanced training in somatic psychotherapy, expressive arts, EMDR, Internal Family Systems, Reiki, and trauma recovery. She has served as a therapist for youth in crisis, a grief and death doula, a music leader, and a guide for countless clients and communities navigating the sacred cycles of birth, death, and rebirth.

Through her sacred brands—Holistic Vibrations, LLC and The Mystic Muse—Tiffany offers trauma-informed healing, intuitive mentorship, and creative direction.

Her body of work includes Mama Crow's Magic, a shamanic healing ministry offering ritual, tarot, and energy medicine, and The Wild Muse Healing Arts Studio, a creative sanctuary for expressive embodiment through voice, movement, and art. She is also the creator of The Lotus: Healing from the Root Up, a trauma recovery program integrating expressive arts, chakra work, ancestral healing, and nervous system regulation.

An eight-time bestselling author, Tiffany's work weaves together psychology, spirituality, and creativity into one integrated path of transformation. She helps others reclaim their voice and purpose through ritual, storytelling, and Spirit-led collaboration, reminding each person of their innate capacity to heal and create.

CONNECT WITH DR. TIFFANY:

Websites: https://www.tiffany-mcbride.org

https://www.themysticmuse.org

Instagram: https://www.instagram.com/witchycrowwmn83

Facebook: https://www.facebook.com/profile.php?id=61552573784401

https://www.facebook.com/profile.php?id=61576753293948

Your DNA is more than data—it's devotion written in light. Each double helix is a hymn of belonging, a sacred geometry.

~ Marilyn Fay

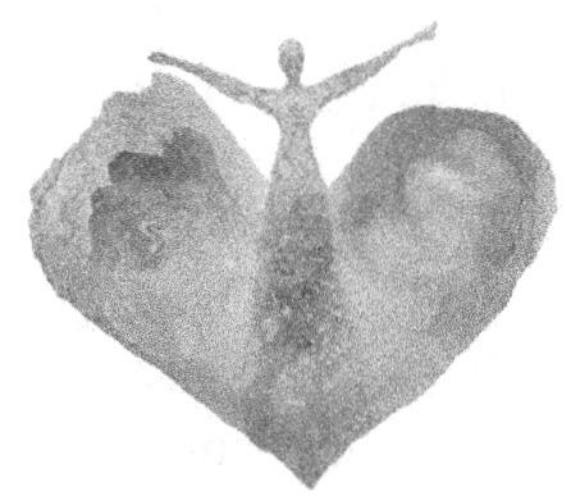

CHAPTER 4

YOUR DNA: DECODE YOUR DIVINE DESIGN
EXPRESS THE ONE-OF-A-KIND CODE WITHIN YOU

Marilyn Fay

INTEGRATIVE HEALING PRACTITIONER

"The privilege of a lifetime is to become who you truly are."
~Carl Jung

MY STORY

DNA testing may be the missing puzzle piece to your mystery symptoms.

My body was in metabolic chaos.

My eyes snapped open in the dark, wide awake.

I glanced over at the clock, 3:00 a.m., again. *How does my body know the exact time?*

This is every night now.

In the morning, I reached for the bathroom faucet and my fingers screamed—swollen, stiff, like someone replaced my joints with rusty hinges overnight.

I reached down to open the bathroom drawer, but couldn't. My shoulder was frozen. *I can't move my arm.* I couldn't brush my hair.

This is all on top of my monthly moon cycles. I mark them on the calendar like preparing for battle. Day one means survival mode, curled up with a heating pad cranked on high, feeling betrayed by my own body. I want to love it—but how do you love what keeps hurting you?

I never thought of myself as a "why me" kind of person—I was the 'everything happens for a reason' girl—and here I am, wondering: *Why me?*

The guilt was almost worse than the pain, missing weeks of my life, plans canceled, fun canceled, moments lost. *I'm in so much pain.* A wave of pain rises from deep inside, through my abdomen, before crashing into a tide of nausea. I brace for the next swell.

The inhaler sits on my nightstand like a lifeline. I need it to breathe. Nobody told me it was depleting my progesterone. Nobody mentioned it's wrecking my hormones. Nobody connected the dots between my inhaler and the hormones that left me in unbearable pain every month.

I became fluent in gaslighting. I learned to minimize my symptoms, to wonder if I was imagining it all. My body kept screaming. I kept dismissing myself.

The doctor glanced up: "Your labs are normal."

Normal. The word that erases you while your body struggles to survive.

I leaned forward. "I can't sleep. As soon as it's time for bed, I'm wide awake. It takes forever to fall asleep, and then I wake up again."

"Maybe try chamomile at bedtime?"

"Can you test my Vitamin D?"

"No, we don't test it because everyone is low." *That makes no sense.*

I sat in my car after, hands gripping the wheel, his words echoing: *Normal.*

If this is normal, what does dying look like?

I am so tired. I want to sleep for ten years.

This sucks! I want to travel. I want to have fun.

How did I get here? This is not the life I planned. I was never sick as a kid. I never missed school.

So, I tried everything—heavy metal detoxes, parasite cleanses, binders, high doses of glutathione and NAC, green juices, and the best supplements. My kitchen counter became a supplement graveyard.

I'm a walking Pinterest board of wellness trends—if it says *detox,* I've tried it twice.

Then came the Nutrigenomics DNA test—how my genes interact with food and nutrients to influence detoxification, metabolism, and energy.

I clicked the PDF while the cursor hovered over it before opening it. Gene variants: CBS, MTHFR, CYP1B1, COMT, PEMT. I see my sulfur-processing genes are stuck. That means I can't break down sulfur foods and supplements like eggs, nuts, seeds, garlic, onions, broccoli, cauliflower, Brussels sprouts, and cabbage—foods I eat all the time. The excess sulfur is toxic, driving inflammation. My estrogen gene creates toxic estrogen metabolites that my body can't clear, explaining the hormonal chaos and the unbearable periods. My detox pathways are blocked—the perfect storm.

The news landed in my body before my mind could catch up, a sharp jolt of truth that left me holding my breath.

"Wow, this makes sense," I whispered. My hand covered my mouth. *I wish I had known all this sooner.*

Every mystery symptom is explained, written in my DNA.

In that moment, I decided to stop forcing my body to heal.

I did everything backward—I introduced detoxes way too early. Took supplements without addressing basic nutrients first and detoxing before opening pathways for toxins to leave.

The DNA test didn't diagnose me—it translated me.

It told me what my body was communicating: *I'm your messenger.*

All I could think was, "I wish I had learned this in high school."

Back then, the idea of mapping our genes was still science fiction.

In 2001, sequencing cost $95 million; by 2007, it cost $1 million, so this simple one-of-a-kind instruction manual was out of reach.

Not anymore.

Now I know every human should know how well they methylate. Methylation affects everything: detoxification, mood, energy, hormones, inflammation, and even how we age. When methylation is disrupted, the body cannot clear waste, hormones, and environmental toxins—like trying to sweep the floor with a broken broom. This knowledge should be foundational—taught in schools, discussed with doctors, and recognized as essential to health.

Your DNA is your unique blueprint, but how it's read depends on you. The environment of your cells—nutrients, stress, toxins, emotions, and lifestyle—shape how your DNA is expressed. Your genetic expression is uniquely yours—the frequency of your authentic self.

Each act of care is cellular reprogramming.

Science calls it epigenetics. I call it the soul's handwriting on the body. You become the author of your own design, the composer of your frequency, the divine in you waiting to be seen all along.

The Tool

Once I understood my DNA, everything changed—but that was only the beginning. Next, I needed to create an environment for my cells where healing could take place. That's why I created Decode the Divine™. This integrative framework helps people understand the language written in their DNA, where biology meets belief and the body becomes a map back to wholeness.

Epigenetics shows that behaviors, thoughts, and surroundings can turn genes on or off—responding to signals from diet, emotion, and environment. Your genes hold the blueprint, but you are the architect.

From this truth, The Awaken Method was born: a constellation of keys designed to create the conditions for your DNA to flourish. Each key reveals what your DNA already knows—only you can be you.

This is where awakening becomes embodied.

This is where science meets soul.

This is The Awaken Method—to decode the divine you.

THE AWAKEN METHOD

Healing isn't a checklist; it's a relationship with your DNA. The Awaken Method isn't meant to be followed rigidly or mastered one key at a time. Think of these as *frequencies* or *doorways*—each one opens a different dimension of your authentic self.

You can move through them intuitively, choosing whichever key resonates most in the moment, or explore them all as a complete experience. Each key nourishes your DNA—reminding your cells you are the architect of your divine design.

Let yourself wander—circle back, mix and match, create your own key. There's no right way—only your way. Let curiosity lead you. Start with whichever key feels alive in this moment.

AWARENESS KEY

Awareness is the foundation for experiencing greater freedom in life. It's the key to recognizing and releasing the emotions, thoughts, and beliefs that limit us, so we can step into the fullness of who we are. Before identity, story, or DNA, there is the silent field of consciousness, the Infinite Being. Awareness is your natural state of being—peaceful, expansive, and free. When you become aware of your inner experience, you reconnect with this deeper truth: you are an infinite being.

Awareness is the unchanging essence of who you are, beyond the fleeting sensations, emotions, and thoughts that come and go. When we become aware of a pattern—a belief, a reaction, a symptom—we step out of identification with it. Awareness is the space that allows transformation to happen.

Awareness is like the sky; thoughts, emotions, and genetic expressions are clouds passing through. The sky never becomes the storm—it simply holds it, allowing it to change shape and dissolve.

Beneath every thought, emotion, and genetic expression is the still field of Infinite Being—consciousness itself, vast and unchanging. When you rest as awareness, you stop identifying with the stories of limitation and begin seeing them as patterns of energy ready to transform.

A simple practice: Pause a few times throughout the day, take a gentle breath, and repeat, "I am awareness." Notice what shifts inside. Awareness is not something you do; it's what you already are.

Mindfulness Key

Mindfulness is the art of returning to the present moment over and over again. It changes your biology and your relationship with life.

Mindfulness shapes your inner environment, the very terrain in which your DNA expresses itself. Each moment of mindful presence reduces stress hormones and activates genes linked to longevity and repair.

Doing one thing at a time rewires the brain. When you interrupt autopilot and choose presence, you carve new pathways.

Practice:

Breathe: Feel the air entering and leaving your body.

Observe: Notice sensations, sounds, emotions, without naming them good or bad.

Engage: Whatever you do—walk, wash dishes, speak—fully participate in the moment.

When you live in a mindful way, you connect your outer life with your inner experience. You become the environment where your DNA thrives.

UPDATING EARLY BELIEFS KEY

Within your sacred DNA lies a living library—a record of every belief, emotion, and decision your soul has made. These early experiences shape your understanding of safety, love, and worth, forming the beliefs through which you see yourself and the world.

Childhood is a period of incredible brain plasticity when the mind operates in an open, receptive state—absorbing beliefs from caregivers, the environment, like a sponge. These early patterns, while once essential for survival, often become outdated as you grow. They may no longer serve the person you're becoming, making it vital to uncover and update them.

One powerful way to access this deep inner intelligence is through a sacred dialogue between your thinking self and your knowing self—the human and the divine spark within.

Here's how to begin:

Take a few slow, gentle breaths and soften into your heart space.

With your dominant hand, write down a question you would like an answer to.

Switch to your non-dominant hand and allow the answer to emerge naturally—without overthinking or judgment. Let your pen move as if it's being guided, allowing words, images, or sensations to arise.

This practice taps into your inner wisdom, the parts of your being that hold wisdom beyond thought. Trust the process and allow this sacred dialogue to unfold. Let your creativity speak.

LOVE KEY

Healing doesn't begin in a supplement bottle or a lab—it begins in the environment you create inside yourself. Love is the frequency that allows your DNA to thrive.

When you love yourself—without finding something wrong or the need to fix—you send a powerful message to every cell: *I love you exactly as you are.* This is the environment that nourishes your DNA.

Research shows that love literally changes the body. It reorganizes chaos, regulates the nervous system, and restores calm. Each act of self-love frees energy that was once trapped in struggle.

A healthy relationship with yourself is the foundation for all others. Love yourself no matter what. How you treat and speak to yourself shapes your well-being—especially when your body feels like it's betraying you. Experiencing pain and dysfunction, it's easy to turn against yourself.

Self-love begins with curiosity and kindness. You're not a single self but a community of parts, each carrying wisdom and purpose. Each part of you has developed to protect or guide you in its own way. When you push pieces of yourself away, the body interprets that rejection as danger, activating survival mode deep in your DNA.

Self-love is being in sync—emotionally, verbally, and energetically. Harsh self-talk keeps the body in an alarmed state, while kindness invites a relaxed healing state for your body.

Some gifts come in tattered wrappings, and your pain is part of your medicine. Know yourself, the story woven through your DNA has already been written.

Practice spending time each day in a feeling you wish to embody, until it becomes your nature.

Love is the most powerful medicine we have.

YOUR VOICE KEY

Your voice is uniquely you. It carries the frequency of your soul and the blueprint of your DNA. It was never meant to stay hidden; it was meant to resonate, be heard, move energy, and touch lives.

No one else has your tone, cadence, or vibration. The world has never heard your exact frequency before, and it never will again. When you speak, sing, or hum from your authentic self, you activate the genetic code of your unique design and awaken the sound of your cellular wisdom. Speak, hum, sing, let your voice move energy.

Authenticity, not perfection, gives your voice strength. The pauses, the nerves, laughter, and even the tears make it real. Your voice doesn't need to be polished or rehearsed; it needs to be true. As you honor your authentic voice, you permit others to do the same. Your truth becomes a tuning fork for the collective, calling others into alignment.

Take five minutes each day to speak aloud. Let your truth move through sound—unfiltered, unpolished, profoundly real—to express the sacred frequency that is you.

SUNLIGHT KEY

Sunlight speaks to your body in its oldest language: light.

Every cell contains mitochondria that awaken in response. Morning sunlight—especially its red and infrared rays—ignites the spark of life, fueling detox and repair.

Long before modern medicine, the sun was the original healer, telling your cells when to wake, rest, and restore. Your mitochondria capture photons and convert them into the fuel that powers every system of your body. Food provides only part of that energy; the majority comes from the sun.

Morning light resets your brain's clock and hormone rhythms—cortisol, melatonin, and thyroid—aligning your body with the natural cycle of day and night. Melatonin protects and restores mitochondrial DNA, scavenging free radicals and repairing damage.

Your DNA is designed to respond to natural cycles of light. Align your biology with rhythms that have guided life for billions of years. This is the oldest form of epigenetic medicine.

Step outside within thirty minutes of sunrise, letting natural light touch your eyes and skin. When you stand in the morning sun, you're not just soaking in warmth—you're remembering what you're made of. You are light.

NOURISH KEY

Nourishment is more than food—it's the care you give to your body, environment, and being part of a community. Nourishment is an ecosystem—a living exchange between you and the world.

We thrive through belonging and meaningful relationships built on shared purpose and faith. Mutual care, laughter, and shared meaning strengthen your immune system and extend longevity—connection nourishes your cells.

Every bite, breath, and thought sends instructions to your DNA. Eat clean, whole foods that support your unique biology, steady energy, and smooth digestion. Choose foods that support life, breathe clean air, and drink pure water.

Reduce your toxic load by noticing what you put on your skin, in your body, and in your home. Avoid inflammatory oils, fake sugars, and plastics that leach harmful chemicals. Simple shifts lighten your body's burden and move you closer to the healing zone.

Remove hidden stressors—toxins, chronic infections, and unprocessed emotions—that drain your energy. Industrial chemicals in our air, water, food, and products have spiraled out of control. Our bodies were never designed to carry this burden, triggering many genetic problems. Give your genes every possible support you can. Choose a "Detox Day" to transform your home: clear expired and highly processed foods, replace toxic cleaners and beauty products, swap plastic containers for glass, and trade harsh laundry detergents that act as endocrine disruptors for non-toxic ones. Use simple ingredients: vinegar, lemon, water, and baking soda.

REST, PLAY, AND MOVEMENT KEY

Your body cannot heal without rest. Sleep is not a luxury; it's medicine. It is the time when your body repairs itself. Deep, consistent sleep restores hormones, supports detoxification, and allows your body to regenerate. This is where your healing takes root and provides the foundation for all healing.

Thriving also requires joy and movement. *What lights you up?* Activities that spark joy—creative, playful, or adventurous—empty your stress bucket and reset your nervous system. Play is not indulgent; it's nourishment for your soul.

Movement is more than exercise; it's how you communicate with your body. Whether walking, dancing, or stretching, your body is designed to move.

Think of your well-being as an energy account. Every restful night, every moment of laughter, and every mindful movement is a deposit. Overwork and worry are withdrawals. In order to thrive, make more deposits than withdrawals. When you honor, rest, play, and move, you create the foundation for your DNA to flourish.

Knowing your DNA allows you to know yourself fully.

You are divinely designed—an infinite being, expansive, vast.

Your DNA is more than data—it's devotion written in light. Each double helix is a hymn of belonging, a sacred geometry.

The invitation of *Decode the Divine*™ is not to fix yourself but to express yourself and the deepest level of your being—to live as the expression of love written in your DNA.

You are both map and message. You are a spark of the divine. Only you can be you—and the world needs the gift of *you:* your presence, your expression, your one-of-a-kind essence. DNA provides the blueprint to be your whole self. Know your DNA. Be you, all the way.

Let's listen. Let's decode.

You are designed on purpose, part of a grand universal design. If your body has been calling for your attention, this is your invitation to listen—with love.

I'd love to create something special for you: a free personalized Guided Meditation Script, uniquely crafted to help you access a relaxed, healing state where you connect with your divine design.

Decode the Divine™ and become the living expression of the light that made you.

Sign up here: https://marilyn-fay.kit.com/dna

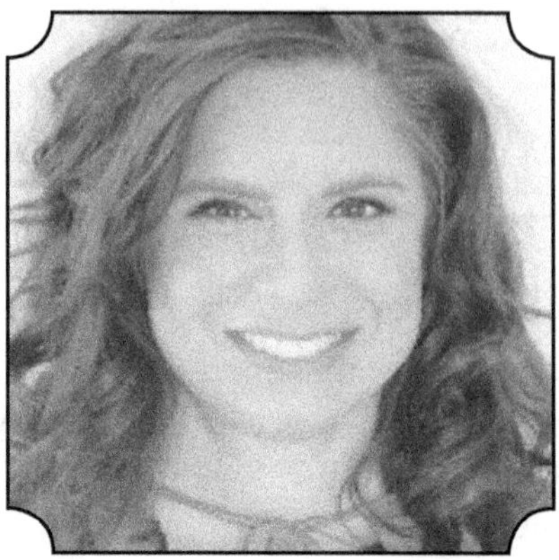

Marilyn Fay is an Integrative Healing Practitioner and founder of Biorhythmic Healing™. She combines nutrigenomics, DNA-based insight, functional lab testing, and mind-body reprogramming to help women transform their health and awaken to their divine design. Through her Decode the Divine™ method, Marilyn helps women in midlife reconnect with their innate power, restoring balance, energy, and confidence by aligning their body's wisdom with their purpose.

After years of unbearable pain, hormone chaos, and sleepless nights, Marilyn discovered the truth written in her DNA—and created a method to help other women do the same.

Her daily mission is to help women shift from confusion about their symptoms to becoming the conscious architects of their genetic expression. She guides clients to decode their unique DNA blueprint, understand why their bodies respond the way they do, and discover what they need to thrive. If you're done with "normal" lab results that don't match how terrible you feel, and you're ready to discover your body's innate instruction manual, Marilyn will meet you exactly where you are—with compassion, wisdom, and a personalized roadmap to healing.

She is a Certified Money Coach, Transformational NLP Practitioner, and Myofascial Release Therapist, weaving the science of epigenetics with the art of embodiment to create whole-person transformation. When she isn't decoding DNA with clients, you'll find her swimming in warm seas, camping under the stars, hosting dinner parties in castles, or curating her next World of Wonder adventure.

CONNECT WITH MARILYN:

Website: http://marilynfay.com/

YouTube: https://www.youtube.com/@marilynfaylemus

Instagram: https://www.instagram.com/biorhythmichealing

Facebook: https://www.facebook.com/profile.php?id=61574955276114

LinkedIn: https://www.linkedin.com/in/marilyn-fay-lemus-b0660b6b

When I look back at those first notebooks full of messy handwriting, circles, arrows, and colored pens, I don't just see data. I see devotion. Those notebooks taught me that health is a language to be learned from the most intelligent system of all - my own body.

~ Caitilin Twain

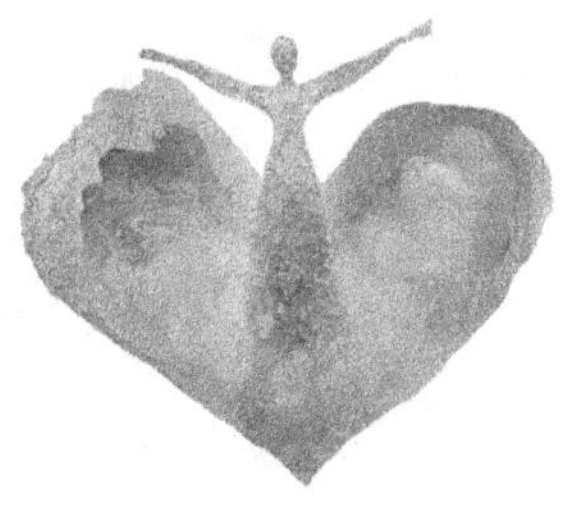

Chapter 5

Listen, Learn, Heal

How Tracking Reconnects You to Yourself

Caitilin Twain

NBC-HWC, HeartMath®, Movement Expert

My Story

I remember the exact moment I hit my breaking point.

I stared at an article claiming that kale, my queen of superfoods, might be to blame for thyroid dysfunctions due to its goitrogenic compounds.

Kale.

The food I practically evangelized to friends and clients. The plant I dutifully grew so I would have a steady supply of raw salads, chips, smoothies, pestos, and soups.

I swore out loud while I laughed from total exasperation, because I *did* have the signs of a slow-functioning thyroid. *Did I make myself sick eating the very thing that was promised to make me healthy?*

This wasn't the first time "health wisdom" turned itself upside down on me. Decades of fighting Lyme disease made me an earnest student of all things health-related. I kept up with the research:

Canola oil was heart-healthy until it wasn't.

Fat was the villain, then sugar was.

Eggs were dangerous, then miraculous.

Butter was banished, then celebrated.

One day, coffee is medicine; the next, it's poison.

Fasting is essential. Fasting is dangerous.

Carbs are good. Carbs are bad.

That kale article was the last straw. I realized I spent years outsourcing my intuition by trusting experts, studies, and even celebrities over the wisdom of my own body, and **I. Was. DONE!**

That day, I reminded myself that we've evolved over millions of years to be brilliant self-healing organisms. So why did I believe that only a special diet or protocol could cure me, especially when all my life experience showed that, in a matter of a few years, they'll likely be proven harmful?

I decided that true healing demands agency. I needed to take matters into my own hands, not out of rebellion, but out of a deep belief that *my body knows how to heal.*

I just had to learn how to listen.

So I took out a blank notebook and wrote on the cover EVIDENCE FROM MY OWN BODY.

I opened to the first page and wrote out my main pain points. I chose three recurring symptoms draining my quality of life: chronic fatigue, brain fog, and joint pain.

Then, underneath those, I listed every possible factor I thought might contribute, either positively or negatively—foods, routines, supplements, even people. Kale made the list, along with caffeine, late-night news consumption, ferments, gluten, and all my supplements.

I didn't know what I was doing. I just knew I needed to start *paying attention.* For the next three months, I logged what I ate, how I slept, how I moved, and how I felt. Patterns emerged.

And there it was: my pain points were consistently worse when I ate raw kale daily. When I cooked it, or skipped it altogether, I felt better.

From then on, I stopped chasing "one-size-fits-all" health advice. I became my own researcher, skeptical of headlines, and committed to testing everything through the lens of my own lived experience. Since then, I've tested countless supplements, protocols, and foods.

The results speak for themselves: the nodules on my thyroid are almost gone without any pharmaceutical intervention. I haven't had a Lyme relapse in over eight years. I'm 54 and have the biomarkers of a healthy 30-year-old.

Tracking did more than improve my health; it changed my relationship with my body. It shifted me from frustration to feeling in control and *deeply* connected to myself.

Over time, my notebook evolved into a tracking system that became a cornerstone of my healing process. Today, it's one of the five pillars of the **C. Twain Method** that I teach to my clients and to other health coaches. It's available to all for free at www.ctwain.com/tracker.

THE TOOL

Tracking replaces generic advice with **personalized data—*your*** data.

It lets you test medications, supplements, protocols, and whatever health fad you're curious about against your genetics, your history, and your current life. It helps you become an expert in your body and make lasting improvements in whatever you want to improve.

Over the years, I've seen extraordinary transformations begin with something as simple as a daily log. Here's why it works.

1. **Awareness Creates Change**

   When you track, you make the invisible visible. You begin to see which foods, behaviors, and emotions bring you balance, and which throw you off. When you see your patterns clearly, you start making better choices, not because you "should," but because you *want* to.

2. Accountability Without Shame

The act of self-tracking instills a sense of accountability and motivation. Knowing that you're monitoring your habits and progress creates a positive feedback loop. I've found that when I'm not tracking, I'm less likely to make the healthier choice, so tracking has become my accountability partner.

3. Collaboration and Clarity

When you bring your tracker to your doctor, you bring data that matters. You can say, "Since doing regular breathwork, I've had only one brief panic attack," or "Over the last three months, my blood pressure average has decreased from 140/100 to 125/82." (I see both these trends on repeat with my clients.) Those specifics lead to responsible medication management. It also shows your doctor that you're an involved and empowered member of your medical team.

4. Connection and Self-Compassion

The hidden gift of tracking is connection. Healing isn't a burden, though there are days when it might feel like that. It's about creating a respectful, cooperative relationship with your body. You begin to understand that your symptoms aren't proof that you're failing; rather, they're messages from your body saying something is wrong.

When you attend to those messages with the same tenderness and patience you would a crying baby, things begin to shift. Every note you write in your tracker is evidence of presence. Every checkmark is an act of care. And eventually, something extraordinary happens! When the body feels seen, the nervous system down-regulates. Pain softens. Sleep deepens. And true, deep healing across all systems occurs.

This isn't magic. It's physiology. Awareness signals safety. Safety unlocks healing.

THE PITFALLS OF TRACKING

Of course, every tool has a shadow side. Tracking can become obsessive when driven by fear rather than curiosity.

Sometimes I see clients treat their trackers like report cards. If they didn't sleep well, they brace for a bad day. If their pain spikes, they see it as a failure rather than the simple feedback it is.

That's not tracking. That's self-surveillance, and it keeps the body locked in stress.

These common traps are easy to fall into:

- **Perfectionism:** Beating yourself up if you didn't log everything perfectly and judging every "setback" as failure. Some clients become "score chasers" with their wearable tech instead of listening to their bodies.

- **Data Overload:** Getting so lost in numbers that you stop noticing how you actually feel. Especially if you're getting data from a wearable like a watch, don't believe the data more than your own experience. Use them to support your self-awareness, not to replace it.

- **Junk Data:** Remember that some data is junk, especially from wearables. Focus on the trends, and let the minutia go.

- **The Nocebo Effect:** Letting one "bad score" or deviation from your "perfect routine" convince you the day is doomed. For example, a bad sleep score might lead to expecting to feel tired all day, and so you will!

Each of these pulls you off the healing path, which is where you feel safe enough to rest, repair, and respond with flexibility.

That's why I teach **compassionate tracking,** which is the practice of collecting data through the lens of self-respect and love, not performance.

How to Track

I highly recommend you download my free tracker at www.ctwain.com/tracker. It comes with a video guiding you through the setup, which may be easier to understand.

Otherwise, make a column on the left side of a page, with just enough room to the right for all the days of the month. Write the month in the top left corner, then all the days of the month. These are the top rows in your tracker.

Under the name of the month, write one to four of your biggest pain points. Maybe it's digestion, energy, and mood. Each pain point gets its own line down the left column. You'll track those daily by assigning them a score (1-10 or 1-5). I like to make this section a graph, with each pain point having its own color.

Under that, add a section for sleep, because sleep impacts everything. Here you can note a sleep score from a tracking device or the hours you slept, including nighttime wakings.

Next, down the left column, list everything you think might be impacting your pain points either negatively or positively. Each day you did/ate/took something, make a note under that day. It might be a simple dot, or you might assign a number to it, e.g., 2 cups of coffee or one glass of wine (those are the cut-off points I found for myself through tracking; more of either will wreck my sleep).

Once a month, step back. What improved? What didn't? What connections between your pain points and potential triggers do you see?

From Data to Dialogue

When I look back at those first notebooks full of messy handwriting, circles, arrows, and colored pens, I don't just see data. I see devotion.

Those notebooks taught me that health is a language to be learned from the most intelligent system of all - my own body. And in the process of that learning, I fell deeply in awe and in love with the brilliant, self-healing organism that I am.

This is what I teach my clients: Your body is not broken. It's communicating.

Tracking is simply interpreting your miraculous system with respectful curiosity.

CLOSING REFLECTION

If you've spent years doing everything "right" and still don't feel well, I want you to know you're not broken. You're simply being invited into a deeper kind of listening.

Start with curiosity. Your body will meet you there.

Curiosity leads to awareness. And awareness through tracking leads to self-connection, self-trust, self-leadership, and excellent health.

When you have those, you'll always know what to do next.

And if you'd like help decoding your body even deeper, whether through advanced technology like continuous glucose monitors or ancient self-healing practices like breathwork, this is the work I do every day with my clients. It would be my honor to guide you into this brilliant landscape.

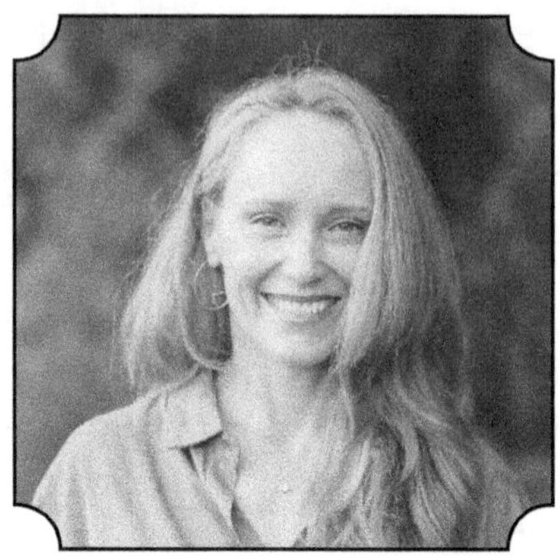

Caitilin Twain is a National Board-Certified Health & Wellness Coach, HeartMath® Trauma-Sensitive Practitioner, Roll Model®, and Movement Specialist who helps people uncover the true sources of pain and illness and restore vibrant health.

After overcoming decades of chronic Lyme disease and a thyroid disorder, Caitilin developed the C.Twain Method - a holistic, science-based, and heart-centered framework built on five pillars: *Mindset, Constructive Rest, Breathwork, Movement & Self-Myofascial Release, and Tracking, Testing & Tech.* Drawing from her early roots as a yoga and breathwork teacher, her work bridges the latest scientific research with ancient wisdom.

Through her private coaching practice, workshops, and retreats, Caitilin helps clients move from confusion to clarity by learning to track what truly matters, release old patterns, and create conditions for the body to heal itself. Her work empowers people to become their own best advocates by uniting data with intuition, self-compassion, and curiosity.

Caitilin teaches clients and fellow coaches how to integrate practical tracking tools and technologies without losing the human heart of coaching. She's known for translating complex science into simple, actionable steps that restore both trust and agency.

Her clients describe working with her as "life-changing," "liberating," and "the missing piece in my healing."

To explore Caitilin's coaching programs, workshops, and free resources, including her signature health tracker featured in this chapter, visit her website below.

CONNECT WITH CAITILIN:

Website: https://www.ctwain.com/

Instagram: https://www.instagram.com/caitilin_twain/

Facebook: https://www.facebook.com/CTwainMethod

LinkedIn: https://www.linkedin.com/in/caitilin-twain-4b823721a/

Through listening to my body and my breath,
I learned to come home to myself and feel safer
staying in my body. A tiny seed of forgiveness
and self-compassion grew. My breath's story
shifted. It was now a companion that stayed with
me to find presence and healing.

~Julianne Thompson Lewis

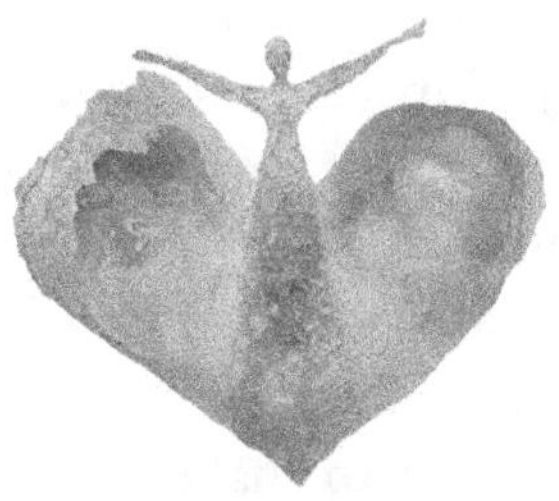

CHAPTER 6

YOUR BREATH HAS A STORY TO TELL
A CREATIVE TOOL FOR LEARNING SAFETY IN YOUR BODY

Julianne Thompson Lewis

M.ED, 200RYT, SOMATIC EXPRESSIVE ARTS PRACTITIONER

"True breathing is like a flower blooming.
If we hold our breath, the bud never opens."
~Chungliang Al Huan

MY STORY

I remember slamming my tailbone on the ice so hard while skating once that it felt like my spine poked my brain. The pain wracked my body and my mind with such force that it knocked the breath right out of me. I held my breath for ten, nine, eight, seven, six, five, four, three, two, one— collapse. Stars swirled around my head.

What I learned as an elite figure skater is that when we fall, we must get back up, keep going, and pretend that the fall had never happened. Put on your mask, straighten up your broken spine, try to catch your breath, and keep going!

This happened so many times throughout my life: falling or being dropped, and never being caught. Every time, I froze like an opossum and held my breath. I pretended that nothing had ever happened, with the hope that nobody would notice.

Eventually, the habit of holding my breath and pretending followed me off the ice and into my marriage, motherhood, and silence. The most frightening moments of freeze I can recall were when my ex-husband and I were deep in the unraveling of our marriage. During what felt like a series of tornado-like arguments that wouldn't quit, I fell into a pattern of bracing for the fall, holding my breath, and leaving my body. During painful, grueling yelling matches, I tried to make sense of his interrogations, our marriage, and our family life with two small boys. I slowly shut down and became almost catatonic, sitting on our bed. All sound around me seemed to fade away as I felt sucked into a black hole. I saw his mouth moving, but couldn't hear or understand what he was saying.

"Julie, where are you? What is wrong with you?" my ex-husband screamed at me. I heard his voice raging, and it snapped me back into the room.

What is wrong with me?
Where did I go?
Why can't I be here?

I forced myself to clasp my clammy hands together and struggled to notice the hard edge of the bed frame pressing into my leg, or the scratchy trim of the comforter stuck underneath me. I searched for the comfort of the family dog, but realized she was hiding at the other end of the house, driven away by the black energy and vacant bodies around her. I knew I was in my bedroom, but it was hard to feel my body and orient myself to the other objects in the room. I couldn't form words or make eye contact with him. I felt lightheaded and sick to my stomach, as if I might faint. There I was holding my breath again. It was as if I could make the world around me stop if I just froze, became invisible, and held my breath until the crisis passed.

Maybe no one will notice I'm here.

I began to recall and take note of all of the moments in life that added up to a pattern of holding my breath: Walking down the aisle of the church at my wedding, terrifying events of sexual assault and objectification, and my first experiences of intimacy in romantic relationships. I starved my brain and body of oxygen so many times that I'd forgotten full conversations, memories, and important dates and anniversaries. The story my breath had been telling me was that it wasn't safe to be me, be seen, or be imperfect.

For so long, I didn't know how to breathe through the difficult moments. I fell, got back up, pretended I never fell, and consequently never learned how to catch myself and recover. Sadly, there wasn't much support during these life events. There were times I asked for help, and times I didn't know how, but no one *picked me up* or offered an arm after each fall.

The pretending and holding became so ingrained into my mind and body's responses to life's stresses that I don't remember actually making a choice to compartmentalize my failures and file them away into a "make-believe vault" of things I hoped nobody would ever find out about me. Like a robot, I masked up and carried on with life, never examining what I might do differently or how I might use my mistakes and failures in life to fail forward.

I reached a day when I could no longer tolerate the holding, disappearing, and pretending that I was keeping up. It became more painful to hold my breath and shut my body down than face the fear of what it meant to stay present, love, and take care of myself. So I had to learn how to catch myself. Slowly, I learned there's nothing wrong with falling or failing. I just never learned the tools or had sufficient support to recover from the falls.

Returning to my creative process was a significant part of my trauma recovery. As a young figure skater, I was very emotive and loved expressing myself on the ice more than completing any difficult jump or spin. I lost myself in letting my body move to the music. I released all the internal pressure and pain, and felt joy and happiness on the ice.

How did I forget this feeling? Where did all of my love for creative expression go?

I immediately sought out therapists specializing in creative arts therapy and devoured every book, workshop, and training I could find. I also started a yoga practice, which taught me the significance of the breath as a life force. Although I continued to meet regularly with a somatic psychotherapist, I noticed the internal shifts when I made art more and more. I wasn't crafting fine art masterpieces. I scribbled, splatter-painted, experimented, and played with paint, fiber, markers, collage, and more. Like a child, I learned my body's creative language all over again.

After every page in my visual journal, I noticed a quieting within. My heart wasn't pounding out of my chest as often. My mind no longer raced like a rollercoaster making loop-de-loops. All the noise and chaos inside began to slow, and gradually I noticed that moments of overwhelm and dissociation became rarer. Feeling my breath return to my body was the healing touchstone for every creative experience.

Through listening to my body and my breath, I learned to come home to myself and feel safer staying in my body. A new appreciation grew for my struggle of disembodiment and dissociation. A tiny seed of forgiveness and self-compassion grew. This felt so tender, like I saw myself as a baby or young child again, and learned to care for her. I witnessed myself working so hard to reclaim presence and the ability to stay. My breath's story shifted. It was now a companion that stayed with me to find presence and healing.

Like moving back into my childhood home, I discovered remnants of old feelings and familiar patterns that brought joy. I let myself play, dance, sing, and lose sense of time in the best way—providing flow and freedom to be me. I clearly outgrew other things. I felt the grief of letting some things go—things that may have served or kept me safe at one time, but now felt old, dusty, and out of place. Perfectionism and people-pleasing gradually felt more uncomfortable and out of alignment with my new way of being *with* myself. Now, when a stressful moment arises, I place my hand over my heart or my belly, take a deep breath in, and let out a big sigh.

> *I am here with you.*
> *You are here, in this moment, with your breath.*
> *We can stay here together.*

I'm finally refusing the mask, and *catching myself as I catch my breath.* My breath has become a gateway back home.

Healing from trauma begins with helping us learn to feel safe in our bodies once again. Over time, listening to your breath and the language of your body can save your life. Ancient yogic perspectives, as well as modern medical research, show that breath practices, also known as *pranayama,* can lower stress levels and bring focus and calm to the mind and body. Breathwork is the fastest way to change the state of our nervous system. Conscious breathing can bring energy to the mind and body when we feel sluggish and foggy, and quiet and calm when we are feeling overwhelmed and flooded with emotion. This down-regulation is an effect of activating the "rest and digest" (parasympathetic) mode of the nervous system. (Schwartz, 2024)

To make the breath's effect more concrete and conscious, we can add a movement practice. In traditional Chinese medicine, the lungs, heart, arms, and hands are deeply connected. "The fingertips conduct circulation of chi (lifeforce or pranayama) into the arms and the trunk (of the body)." (Little, 2016). For many people in trauma recovery, large muscle movements may feel too scary and vulnerable. So we can start small, by integrating simple mark-making practices with conscious breathing.

The Tool

Your own breath has a story to tell, also. This story will reflect back to you, your experience, and if you listen carefully, it can teach you to slow down and develop greater self-compassion. A visual expression of your breath can reveal its color, texture, movement, and temperature, like biofeedback. Over time, the practice will help you notice when you're holding, and it'll become more familiar to *touch* your breath to bring you back home.

I recommend reading through the instructions a couple of times before you try the full practice. Gather some plain, unlined paper, colored pencils, oil pastels, markers, or watercolor paints with brushes and a small cup of water. Find a comfortable and supportive chair to sit in, and keep the art materials easily accessible next to you.

If it's comfortable, close your eyes or soften your gaze to a fixed point. Press the soles of your feet into the floor, draw a breath in through your nose, as you lengthen your spine and reach upward with the crown of your head. As you exhale through your mouth, feel your spine against the back of the chair and intentionally drop your shoulders down your back. Notice your seat in the chair. Continue to consciously connect with your breathing for several more rounds of inhalations and exhalations, finding a natural rhythm. There's no need to change or analyze anything about your breath, just notice without judgment.

Begin gently bringing your awareness to where you notice the air entering and leaving your body. If you like, you can place a hand on the areas of the body where you notice the inhalation and the exhalation. If touch isn't feeling good, try to stay with the awareness of your breath; in through your nose, and out through your mouth slowly, like you're slowly blowing out a candle.

As you observe your breath, imagine yourself like a curious bee investigating a delicate flower. Does your breath have a color, a shape, movement, or texture? Is it warm, cool, soft, rough, fast, or slow? Be careful not to get caught in the story about why your breath may be a certain way. If you catch yourself going there, gently invite yourself back, encouraging yourself to stay curious and observant of your breath.

After eight to ten breaths, crack open your eyes and choose a drawing or painting tool that reflects the color of your breath. Let the inhales and exhales begin to flow out of your body, through your hand, and onto the paper. As you continue tuning inward, give yourself permission to choose different art mediums and colors. Ask your breath again if it's moving fast or slow, or in a specific pattern, and let yourself move the marks intuitively over the paper.

It can be tricky to trust yourself with this process without falling into a controlled or planned design or pattern. Just imagine your breath moving its way through your hand and around the paper intuitively. You may see something emerge on the paper that entices you to repeat a motion, color, pattern, or texture. Let your attention follow that as well. You could imagine that you are drawing a portrait or a landscape of your breath.

You can experiment with trying this process with your eyes closed, or with your non-dominant hand, which has the added benefit of creating more mindfulness and presence, and aids in helping you get in touch with the more emotional side of creative exploration. It can also help you bypass the more critical, conscious, and logical side of your brain and help you access your unconscious. Using your non-dominant hand challenges your brain, leading to better communication between both hemispheres and the creation of new neural pathways.

Over time, see what noticing and expressing your breath is like in moments when you don't have your art materials handy. Maybe sitting at a stoplight in stressful traffic, or waiting in a doctor's office for a procedure or an appointment. Notice your breath and gently slow down the inhalations and exhalations. Then, using your pointer finger, "draw" your breath on your other hand, your leg, a table, or the air. Name out loud (or quietly in your head) the colors, shapes, movements, and patterns you notice your breath taking.

Remember that learning to notice and listen to our breath takes time and practice. Try to be kind and patient with yourself, as if you were supporting a good friend through this process. There is no *wrong* way to do this practice. It's simply an evolving conversation with your breath and your body, listening closely to your breath's story and responding to it with support, like you would with a dear friend. The breath is deeply connected to our emotions, and you may notice big emotions arise during the practice. If you feel overwhelmed, pause and look around the room, ground your feet, and notice the feeling of the chair supporting you. Slowly return to the practice when you're ready.

My wish for you is to develop a relationship with your breath, which serves as a gauge of your internal state and a signal that can help direct you back toward your inner landscape to find a sense of *homecoming*. As you discover this forgotten terrain, let yourself marvel in the preciousness that is human breath. For an audio version of this guided practice and more resources, find me at CreateMindBody.com.

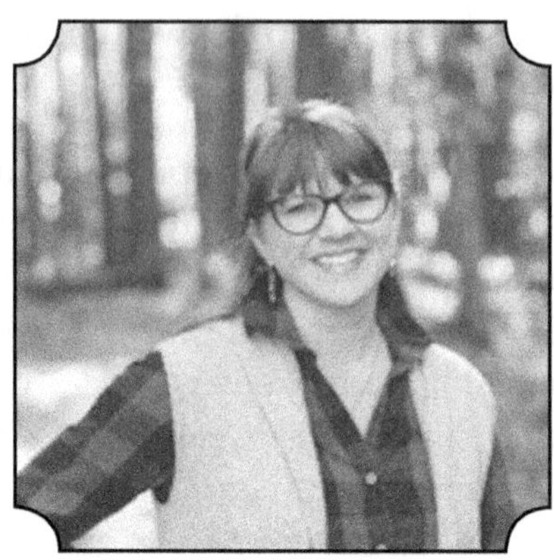

Julianne Thompson Lewis, M.Ed., is a New York State licensed educator and a 200-hour RYT. She has trained with Dr. Ann Biasetti in yoga therapeutics, interoception, and somatic awareness; received certification in Applied Polyvagal Theory in Therapeutic Yoga for Trauma Recovery, and is in the process of certification in Mindful Awareness in Body-Oriented Therapy (MABT), a somatic trauma recovery protocol developed by researcher and trauma recovery practitioner Dr. Cynthia Price. As a therapeutic yoga instructor, Julianne enjoys sharing the powerful practices of yin and restorative yoga, along with breathwork and embodied expressive arts. She is also a co-founder of C.R.E.A.T.E. Community Studios, a non-profit organization making therapeutic expressive arts affordable and accessible to ALL ages and abilities in the Capital Region of New York. Julianne is excited to share her experience and knowledge of the deeply healing connections between yoga, creative arts, and a healthy nervous system.

REFERENCE LIST:

Schwartz, Arielle. 2024. *Applied Polyvagal Theory in Yoga: Therapeutic Practices for Emotional Health.* Norton Professional Books

Little, Tias. 2016. *Yoga of the Subtle Body: A Guide to the Physical and Energetic Anatomy of Yoga.* Shambhala Publications

CONNECT WITH JULIANNE:

Website: https://createmindbody.com/

Email: juliecreatemindbody@gmail.com

Instagram: http://www.instagram.com/createmindbody

Facebook: https://www.facebook.com/CreateMindBodyWellness

Wise boundaries are vital for safe, effective functioning and relate to all aspects of life. They include physical, cognitive, and emotional limits that protect our health, time, relationships, finances, and energy.

~Rev. Dr. Karen Schuder

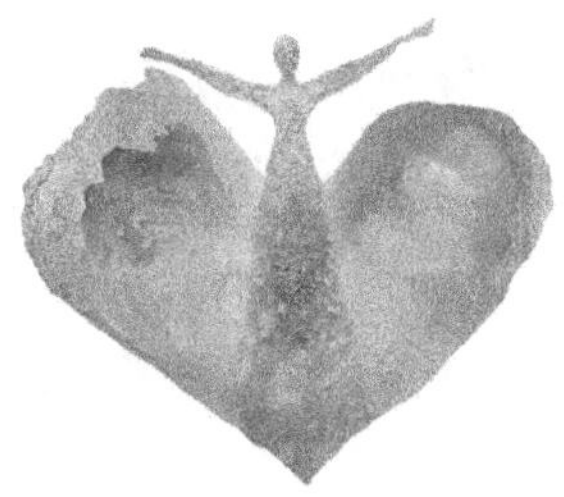

CHAPTER 7

INCREASE INNER PEACE
PROMOTE HEALTHY LIMITS AND THE COURAGE TO SAY "NO"

Rev. Dr. Karen Schuder

EdD, MDiv, MAM

MY STORY

"You are so beautiful," Ned said while caressing my hand. He was the head of staff where I was doing a professional internship. He continued, "I'm lonely. I think you're smart and I enjoy being with you."

What?! I'm married and he knows that! My heart rate accelerated while internal alarms rang loudly. The classroom's colorful posters and empty chairs faded into the background as the meeting jumped into unknown territory. I quickly pulled my hand away while sliding the chair back with a loud screech.

My mind screamed "no," but my throat tightened and I remained silent. As soon as he finished talking, I dashed from the room. Without stopping to grab my coat, I ran home to my husband and infant son, thinking:

He's my boss, what do I do?
I feel gross.

Never be alone with him again.
Will he punish me for reacting negatively?
I'm so ashamed.
Do I tell someone? Do I tell my husband?
Is this what professional life looks like?

I burst through our apartment door. Steve, who sat on the floor with our son and an array of colorful toys, looked up quickly.

"What's wrong?" he asked.
What do I say? Where do I start?

My workday included a variety of challenges. I endured listening to colleagues' complaints, learned about responsibilities added to my position, and attended unexpected meetings. On top of this growing workload, I was the primary caregiver for our son, supported Steve in his demanding career, and had coursework to keep up with. Ned's behavior tipped me over the edge.

Tears sprang forth as I dropped to the floor and threw my arms around Steve. He tightened his arms around me, kissed me on the cheek, and said,

"It's okay. You're okay now. What's going on?"

"I had a meeting with Ned." I took a deep breath to calm myself and explained, "He caressed my hand and said things like 'You're so beautiful and I want to be with you.' I feel so bad. I am so sorry."

"What are you sorry about? You did nothing wrong. How can I help you?"

"Just hold me and tell me you still love me."

"I love you."

A few days later, I walked into the building with my head held high, having convinced Steve to let me handle my work challenges.

I can do this.
Make sure you are never in a room alone with Ned, and only talk with him when necessary. If he does anything inappropriate, say "No!" and turn

in your resignation.
What if. . .Nope, I'm not going to go there.
I should have said, "NO!" before, but now I'm prepared.
I can do this.

My internship continued without a need to confront Ned. I made sure I was never alone with him and let him know I was uncomfortable with his previous comments. I also considered time and energy constraints. I needed to be proactive about what I took on, including my colleagues' attitudes. When asked to lead a new class or meeting outside my job description, I considered the request rather than automatically saying "yes." Sometimes I said, "No."

Society taught me it's impolite to say "no." I wanted to please people and succeed, which increased the difficulty of promoting healthy boundaries. When faced with other people's needs and a lack of healthy limits, my mental narrative often got in the way.

I want to make them happy.
I need to impress to succeed.
I feel selfish focusing on my own needs.
Am I overreacting?

During my internship, I experienced the chaos, dysfunction, and burnout associated with a lack of healthy limits and the inability to say "no." Limits are boundaries that clarify what we are and aren't responsible for. They help us understand what we need to be concerned about and what we can let go of.

THE IMPORTANCE OF BOUNDARIES

Wise boundaries are vital for safe, effective functioning and relate to all aspects of life. They include physical, cognitive, and emotional limits that protect our health, time, relationships, finances, and energy. Taking time to walk and enjoy family, saving money for a trip, or saying "no" to a request all reveal limits. So does refusing to be alone with someone who violated our trust. Boundaries honor individuality and allow us to connect with others in healthy, sustainable ways.

Consider the importance of boundaries during my internship. Frequent responsibility changes, ongoing exposure to other people's discontent, and Ned's inappropriate behaviors amplified the need for limits. Not long after I left, organizational conflict erupted and allegations surfaced regarding Ned's misconduct. I learned an important lesson: We need to advocate for our own well-being and this includes fostering healthy limits.

Promoting boundaries isn't selfish. Limits increase positive connections and our ability to help others. They counter burnout while expanding inner peace and resilience. Despite this, many individuals and organizations fail to honor healthy boundaries. A lack of understanding or respect doesn't negate the need for limits. When we see boundaries as a negative, we risk putting ourselves in danger or taking on more than what is viable, including other people's emotions.

WHAT ARE WE EMOTIONALLY RESPONSIBLE FOR?

As I provided support for unhappy colleagues or faced Ned's loneliness, was I responsible for taking care of their emotional needs? When exposed to other people's discontent, anxiety, sadness, or suffering, are we responsible for fixing how they feel? No. We can provide support and encouragement, but we're only responsible for our own emotions.

We aren't accountable for other people's emotional well-being. I could let go of the guilt and shame attached to an inability to change others' lives. I related to Ned's loneliness, but didn't need to feel responsible for changing it. Learning this allowed me to let go of anxiety and find the courage to say, "No." We often equate caring with taking on and 'fixing' others' emotional health, but this isn't realistic. Healthy boundaries honor that we each have our own emotional journey.

Emotional boundaries are important for personal and professional relationships, especially when suffering is involved. I know setting limits is hard with people we're close to, but they're still vital. We lose perspective more quickly when our child is sobbing, our husband is stressed, or our parents are ill. However, we risk our own health and cannot effectively help others when we lose emotional distinctiveness.

Clarifying the distinction between empathy and compassion can help us understand what we're emotionally responsible for. Empathy, in its original Greek, means to feel what others feel. It helps us connect, but we must keep empathy in perspective, or we give up too much of ourselves.

Empathy fosters compassion, which is defined as the awareness of suffering accompanied by a desire to end it. This honors emotional boundaries. We are each responsible for our own emotions and should allow others to experience theirs and take responsibility for them. We can care about others, try to alleviate suffering, and still experience the joys of our own emotional journeys.

Promoting healthy boundaries is easier said than done. Awareness is an important step towards honoring wise limits. You can foster inner peace and the courage to say "no" with practical strategies for discerning and setting limits.

THE TOOL

LIST BOUNDARY BENEFITS

A great starting point is to consider how healthy boundaries will benefit you and others. Think about an individual or group you want to establish healthy boundaries with. Write a list of the benefits to show that promoting limits is advantageous for everyone involved.

A list may include:

- My relationships will be more sustainable and enjoyable.

- I'll be able to take care of myself.

- I'm more likely to experience and share hope.

- We can know better who will do what.

- We'll better remember our responsibilities.

- We'll find our time together more meaningful.

- I will feel safer.

- I'll have more energy to help and deal with challenges.

- I can be more authentic.

- I can allow others to be more authentic and express how they're feeling without it bothering me as much.

- I can say "no" when I don't feel right about something.

- We will be able to function more effectively.

You can use statements from your list to explain how a boundary promotes everyone's well-being. Change is difficult, so be prepared for questions and opposition. Promoting healthy limits does not give us license to be disrespectful or unkind, but does mean we need to be able to say "no." Awareness of the positives will provide courage and inspiration when someone challenges efforts to establish boundaries.

CLARIFY RESPONSIBILITIES

We often sense we need to do something different to promote wellbeing and wise limits, but the "what" can be murky. We may often feel tired, get crabby more easily, or lose a sense of hope. We get caught up in other people's emotions and miss out on the joys of our own lives. We know this isn't how we want to live, but we don't understand how to change. Clarifying our responsibilities helps us identify what boundaries can assist and how to implement them.

Creatively clarify responsibilities by using a yard or garden metaphor. On a piece of paper, draw a large square in the middle surrounded by other squares. (You can find an example on my website.) The center square is your yard or garden and represents what you're responsible for. Neighboring squares identify other people's yards and responsibilities.

Consider what you're responsible for. Refer to job descriptions and household duties, but also include your physical, cognitive, emotional, social, and financial health. Personal well-being should be at the top of your list. Our emotions also rank high. Remember, self-care is not selfish. Healthy people can connect with and help others more effectively. A complete list of responsibilities includes what we are obligated to provide for ourselves.

Write your responsibilities inside the center square. Have fun and decorate it with joyful flowers or wise trees. Include pesky weeds you do not desire but must take care of. Use colors and shapes to personalize your yard. Make sure the space shows what you're responsible for.

After clarifying your responsibilities, identify other people's responsibilities. Designate surrounding yards for those you regularly interact with. This may include people you care for, family members, friends, coworkers, or colleagues. Write some responsibilities in their squares, such as attitude, health, and emotions. We recognize people's individuality and ability to be responsible by honoring their obligations.

What responsibilities in other people's yards do you tend to take on? Or what obligations in your yard do other people take on? It's too easy to assume other people's responsibilities when we're helpers or want to impress. Despite good intentions, spending too much time in other people's yards promotes unsustainable relationships. We unintentionally communicate, "You can't handle this," when repeatedly assuming other people's responsibilities.

Choose practical ways to take care of your responsibilities without taking on other people's duties. Determine what you can let go of, especially guilt or shame. Decide when you need to say, "No." Consider what life looks like when you're thriving. Include values and purpose to reflect what's important. Write down some limits to help you spend more time in your yard and thrive even while helping others during difficult times.

Remember, your efforts aren't selfish and will benefit everyone involved. Be patient and persistent. It may seem easier to leap into other people's yards, especially when anxiety is present. The following strategy can help you promote inner peace and the courage to say "no" by encouraging emotional differentiation amid other people's anxiety and emotions.

MAINTAIN EMOTIONAL INDIVIDUALITY

Emotional differentiation helps us experience our journey as we interact with and care for others. We can remain calm and allow others to express their feelings when we distinguish between our emotions and theirs. A simple strategy to promote this involves picturing an energy field around each person.

Imagine a bubble around individuals whose emotions affect you. Envision your bubble and remember who you are. Think of a message you can use to promote emotional differentiation, such as "I am (name), I care, and I can feel differently." Imagine the emotional bubbles and remember your message when feeling anxious during an encounter. Other people will affect us, but we can influence how they affect us.

My internship experiences with colleagues, including Ned, weighed on me until I remembered what I was and wasn't responsible for. I allowed myself to let go of the guilt and shame connected to other people's attitudes and behaviors. This gave me peace and the courage to say "no." I learned from my responses and focused on my own emotional journey. Limits enabled me to heal, support others, and experience the simple joys of my own life.

Understanding and promoting healthy boundaries takes time, but it's well worth the effort. Limits help us increase inner peace, wisdom to know when to say "no," and the courage to do so. They're not selfish or rude, but make the world a healthier place. I hope you find much peace and courage as you let go of what isn't yours to carry. Each time you foster a healthy boundary, you proclaim an essential reality: Your well-being is important.

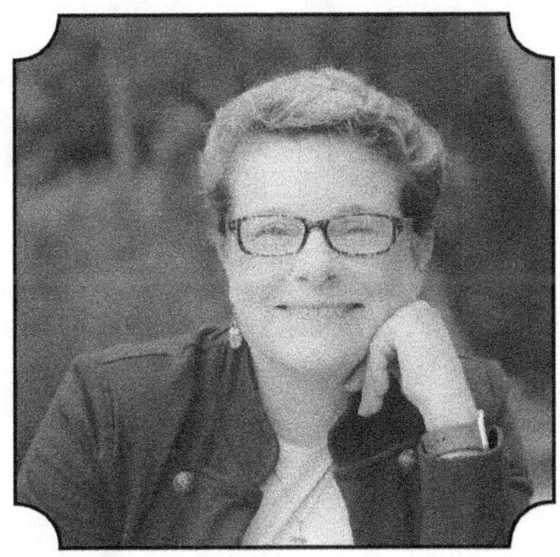

Karen Schuder, international best-selling author and speaker, has extensive experience promoting resilience, inner peace, and role sustainability. Years of helping people during traumatic times, leading organizations, and working globally inform her work with people in personal and professional helping roles.

Karen offers life-changing concepts and practical strategies with an enjoyable, interactive approach. Her book is a valuable resource for helping you promote life balance, inner peace, and resilience with healthy boundaries, self-compassion, purpose, and other topics. Check out her book or website for more strategies!

This chapter includes information and excerpts from Karen's book *Resilient and Sustainable Caring: Your Guide to Thrive While Helping Others,* published by Whole Person Associates, and her chapter "Promote Healthy Boundaries to Thrive: Create Balance for Resilient and Sustainable Caregiving" in *The Caregiver's Advocate: A Complete Guide to Support and Resources,* published by Brave Healer Productions.

Learn more about Karen's work and how to promote life balance characterized by healthy boundaries, resilience, positivity, and decreased anxiety.

CONNECT WITH KAREN:

Website: https://www.karenschuder.com/

Wisdom is the gold that remains after everything
false has burned away.

~Rev. Dr. Ahriana Platten

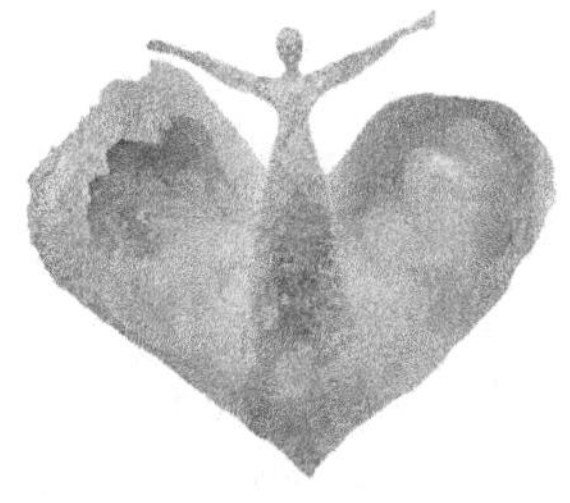

Chapter 8

Harvesting Wisdom
How Menopause Turns Pain into Power

Rev. Dr. Ahriana Platten

The patriarchy fears this part for a reason.

My Story

Menopause didn't creep in quietly. It rose like a storm at sea. The air thickened, the tide of my own body turned, and everything I thought I knew about myself began to change. Sleep was lost in swells of overthinking. Anger rolled through me like lightning, ready to strike. I fell into waves of panic, heart pounding, and cold sweat, meeting the question, "What's happening to me?"

My body answered with silence first, then with a roar that came from a place deeper inside than I knew possible. It wasn't anger at anyone in particular. It was the sound of a lifetime of suppressed rage.

My life has always been full. I've experienced love that opened galaxies inside me and raised children who grew into wise souls. I've enjoyed sacred work, a sense of purpose, and the satisfaction of serving. Yet beneath all the good in my world, lives a quieter story, one I've conveniently stored in a dark corner of my heart. For most of the first half of my adult life, it huddled there, not-so-patiently waiting for the experience of menopause to set it free.

This is the story of the young woman I used to be. The one who learned too early how much love could hurt. The one who smiled when she wanted to scream because it was safer that way. The one who believed that silence was strength. The one who'd been cursed, abused, and made to feel that being a woman meant she would always be "less than."

I remember the first night the memories hunted me down. I sat on the edge of my bed, sweating through an unexplainable tremor of anxiety, when I heard myself speak out loud, "I can't do this." And somewhere inside, a small voice replied, *Then don't.*

Instead of pushing that voice back down, I allowed images to open deep inside, entering my conscious mind. I welcomed memories I hadn't entertained in decades. Faces appeared. Ones I'd buried in forgiveness I didn't really feel. The mind of my younger self emerged trying to make sense of what happened back then, but all she could come up with was, "It must have been my fault."

No, sweetheart. It was never your fault. You were trying to love people who didn't know how to love themselves, or anyone else, for that matter.

The tears came. Not the neat, quiet kind, but the kind that came in wild, body-shaking torrents. I wept for that girl. I wept as that girl.

You're safe now. You can stop pretending. I told her

She didn't believe me at first.

For years, I carried an old belief that something inside me was broken, and I built my life around that mistaken truth. I turned it into achievements, caretaking, and strength. I made it look like wisdom when it was really survival. Menopause stripped away the disguise.

The fire in my body kept rising, wave after wave. An inner knowing informed my understanding that it wasn't punishment. It was purification.

Every flush of heat was an ancient cleansing. Every panic attack was a summons to remember.

One morning, after another restless night, I looked at my reflection and thought, *This has to mean something. It's too powerful to be happening for no reason.*

The woman in the mirror nodded. She inherently knew.

Menopause dredges the riverbed of our lives, stirring what has long settled at the bottom. Old griefs, forgotten fears, and the echoes of our earliest wounds rise to the surface. It's not cruelty or some strange torture imposed on women by the universe that brings up these wounds. It's grace. Like a plant that blooms only once in a lifetime, this midlife blossom unfurls from the deep roots of experience, releasing the fragrance of healing and self-knowledge. What once felt like pain reveals itself as the dark soil in which wisdom grows, rich with the nutrients of truth. The heat of this passage softens what was hardened, opens what was hidden, and invites us to gather the gifts our younger selves couldn't yet see.

It took months before my rage softened into clarity, and years before I began to speak differently, to move differently. I stopped apologizing for my feelings. When someone crossed a line, I said so. When I needed rest, I rested. When I needed silence, I chose it.

I recall a conversation with my best friend that brought powerful insight.

"Do you miss who you used to be?"

I thought about it for a moment, then heard myself say, "No. I feel like I'm meeting the woman I was born to be, but I couldn't reach her until everything in my inner psyche burned down."

That's when I finally began to understand how misinformed we are. This fire, this reckoning, this transformation is holy. Western culture teaches women to dread menopause. Society barely speaks the word and buries a powerful truth in lies about aging. We've been taught to feel shame for the changes we go through rather than learning that menopause has the potential to unlock our greatest wisdom. When we stop carrying the midlife stories imposed upon us, we can't help but realize that menopause isn't madness, it's metamorphosis.

And yes, the patriarchy fears that awareness, because you can't convince a wise woman that she's anything less than wise.

But wisdom takes time to gather. Some evenings, the room fell into that deep, forgiving silence only candlelight understands. I struck a match, and the flame flickered awake, small and steady. My palm rested over my heart, warm against the pulse that carried me through everything. "Show me," I whispered. The air changed. Memories began to move, slow and shapeless, rising like smoke curling from the wick. A slammed door. A name I hadn't spoken in years—a tremor in my chest where old fear still lived. I didn't turn away. I stayed, breathing through the ache, letting each ghost speak until it grew soft enough to rest. Healing came in small, steady acts of courage. The courage to stop blaming myself. The courage to look in the mirror and say, "I forgive you." The courage to be still when I once would've powered through.

I journaled about it all. I wrote letters to my younger self at different ages and in different situations, each one a love note to the girl who didn't know she was born sacred. When I finished writing, I buried those letters deep in the crevices between rock formations at a mountainous park near my home, releasing the pain to the earth so that something new could grow.

Menopause didn't destroy me; it revealed me. Beneath the layers of fear and duty was a woman who no longer needed to please, prove, or hide. A woman who could love without losing herself. The anger that once frightened me became clarity. The tears became release. The heat became my fire, my own holy flame of transformation. I realized the story I carried, the one about being somehow broken, was never true. The harm done to me never defined me. What defined me was my own self-judgement, and, over time, what healed me was my own self-love.

Menopause changed my relationship with truth. It stripped away illusion, leaving only what was real. And what was real was remarkable.

Wisdom is the gold that remains after everything false has burned away.

THE TOOL

To heal the wounds that menopause brings into the light is a journey into tenderness, courage, and ritual. The practice I offer here honors the body as the temple of transformation and helps turn pain into power. It invites you to meet yourself where you are, with breath, body, and flame as your allies. If you're anything like me, you'll do this exercise more than once.

STEP ONE: CREATE A SANCTUARY

Choose a space where you can be alone and uninterrupted. Dim the lights or go outdoors if possible. Light a candle or small fire. Let it symbolize the sacred flame within you, the heat that transforms. Bring a journal, a pen, and something natural to represent yourself, perhaps a stone, feather, or flower. Sit quietly. Feel your breath moving through you. Let the light steady you. You're safe here. You are sacred.

STEP TWO: NAME WHAT WAS HIDDEN

Close your eyes and place your hand on your heart. Ask your body, "What memory or belief is ready to be released?" Trust whatever arises. It might be a word, an image, or a sensation. Be patient until it comes to your mind and heart. Don't overanalyze it. Simply listen. When you're ready, write it down. Be specific and honest. If tears come, let them. They're part of the cleansing. This step invites you to see your truth clearly and to speak the unspoken, giving voice to what was once silenced.

STEP THREE: OFFER IT TO THE FLAME

Read your words aloud, beginning with, "I release. . ." and then add what you've written. Speak slowly, as if giving this burden to the fire for purification. As you watch the flame flicker, imagine the old pain dissolving into smoke.

"What was once my wound now becomes my wisdom."

Let the smoke carry your offering upward, transforming hurt into the breath of the Holy. Notice how your body feels as you let go. You may sense warmth in your chest, a deep breath, or a softening in your belly. These are signs of release.

STEP FOUR: CALL BACK YOUR POWER

Now, take your symbolic object (the stone, feather, or flower) and hold it in your palms. Breathe into it and say, "I reclaim all the power I gave away. I bring home every part of myself that was lost." Feel warmth moving through your hands, your arms, your chest. Imagine that warmth anchoring into your belly, your center of strength. The act of reclaiming isn't about taking from others. It's about remembering that your essence was never truly lost. Your power has always lived inside you, waiting for your permission to return. Later, after the ceremony, place the item where you can see it so you remember the work you've done.

STEP FIVE: LISTEN FOR THE GIFT

Sit quietly again. Ask your inner wisdom, "What have I learned from what I've lived through?" Let words, images, or sensations come. Write them down without judgment. These are the seeds of your wisdom harvest. You might be surprised by what arises. Many women experience a new sense of compassion, clarity, and confidence.

The lessons you harvest from pain are the very medicine you came here to carry. Allow yourself to recognize that, even in your hardest moments, your life has been your greatest teacher.

STEP SIX: SEAL THE HEALING

When you feel complete, say aloud: "I honor the woman I was, the woman I am, and the woman I am still becoming. All are sacred. All are one." Extinguish the candle with a breath of gratitude. Feel the stillness that follows. The healing continues long after the flame is gone. It works its way through your thoughts, your body, your relationships, and your choices. You've marked this moment as sacred, and sacredness has a way of rippling outward.

LIVING THE WISDOM

This practice requires more than one night by the fire. It invites you to learn to live from your inner flame every day. When anger rises, see it as your protector, signaling that something needs to change. When sadness surfaces, let it soften you rather than undo you. When heat floods your body, breathe into it and ask it to, "Burn away what is not mine."

This is how pain becomes power, not by erasing the past, but by transforming your relationship to it. As women, we're trained to minimize our discomfort, to apologize for our emotions, to make ourselves palatable. But menopause teaches a different lesson. It says, "Stop shrinking. Stop pleasing. Begin embodying." Each time we choose truth over silence, we heal. Each time we rest instead of hustling, we reclaim balance. Each time we forgive ourselves, we return to love.

Our bodies know what the mind forgets: that every ending is also a beginning. The notion that menopause is the loss of youth is a lie. Yes, your body changes. Every bit of you changes mind, body, and spirit. Menopause is the unveiling of the wise woman, and she's very different from who you've been. The wise woman is done bending her knee. She stands in her knowing and speaks with the voice of experience rather than fear. When you walk through this fire consciously, you emerge changed. While it's true that few of us come out of menopause unscathed, when we do the work available to us, we come out as the wisdom-keepers the world needs now.

The Wise Woman is born from deep excavation and tenacity. She carries her history as holy text, her scars as scripture, and her truth as her torch.

So, dear reader, light your candle. Sit with your story. Harvest your truth. Let the fire remind you that nothing about you is broken. The heat within you signals your initiation into the wisdom years, and now is the time to come into your power.

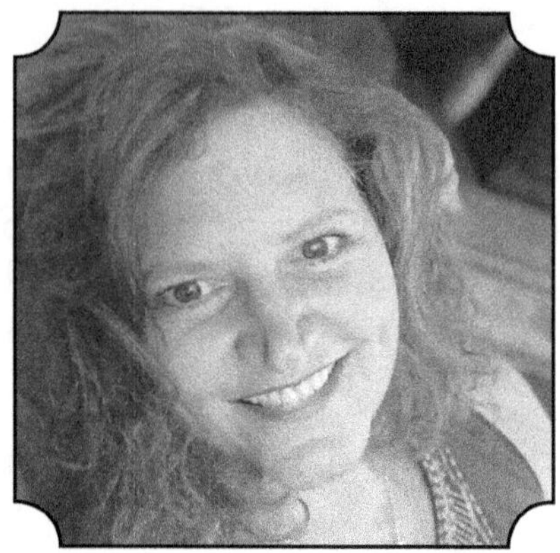

Rev. Dr. Ahriana Platten believes the world changes when women remember their power. Fiercely loving and deeply devoted to the sacred, she's an ordained minister who served as an Ambassador for the Parliament of the World's Religions. She's a featured wisdom-keeper in the documentary series "Time of the Sixth Sun" and the founder of A Soulfull World, a global wisdom community reaching people in more than 50 countries. She's the author of *Sacred Menopause: A Woman's Guide to Sovereignty,* where you can find more tools, ceremonies, and guidance for moving through women's midlife mysteries. Through her teaching, writing, and global work, Ahriana invites women to reclaim their voice, their intuition, and their joy. She blends ancient wisdom with modern reverence, teaching us how to fully embody and express the indwelling Divine. Whether she's leading a circle, blessing a new beginning, or laughing with other wise women, she calls forth the understanding that when one woman rises, we all rise.

Connect with Ahriana:

Menopause classes & retreats:
http://www.asoulfullworld.com/sacredmenopause

Spiritual Training & Mentoring: http://www.asoulfullworld.com

Facebook: https://www.facebook.com/ahriana.platten

Instagram: https://www.instagram.com/ahriana_platten/

LinkedIn: https://www.linkedin.com/in/ahriana-platten/

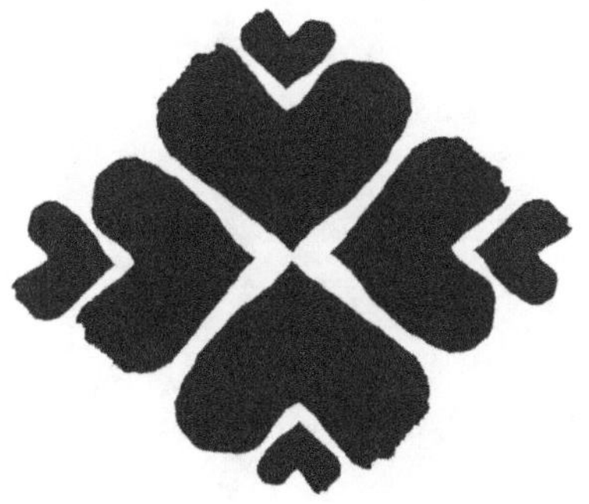

PAIN RELIEF

When we walk with chronic pain and not against it,
rhythm is the path, renewal is the doorway, and
reverence is the key.

~ Jean Voice Dart

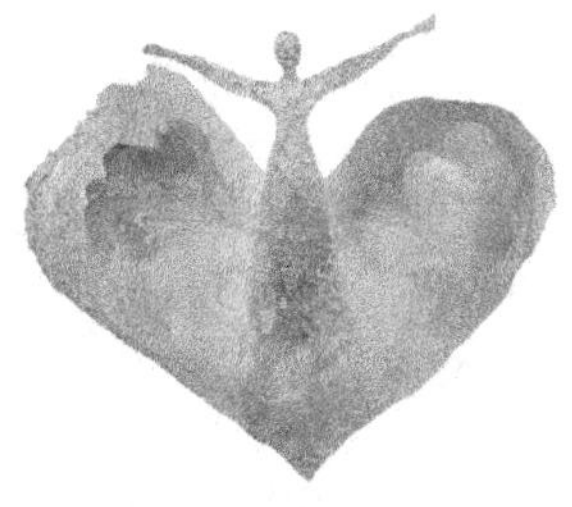

CHAPTER 9

From Ache to Awake
Beating Pain with Rhythmic Renewal and Reverence

Jean Voice Dart

Expressive Arts Psychotherapist

"When we walk with chronic pain and not against it, rhythm is the path, renewal is the doorway, and reverence is the key."
~ Jean Voice Dart, MS, RMT

My Story

Rhythm is my medicine, the heartbeat of family, the pulse of belonging, and the breath of grace. It's not just movement or sound; it's vital to my existence.

The bentwood rocker creaks like a hymn. Its rhythm teases me with a heartfelt yearning. I hold my infant son against my chest, his breath syncing with mine. I hum as his heartbeat echoes a melody—a gentle lullaby born from within.

"I'm scared," I whisper. "Thank you for being here."

"Mmm-mm-mm," he hums.

"Being scared is a good thing." My eyes widen, and I smile with joy. "It means it's time to try something new."

"Gahglag coo!" The gurgling sound bursts through his lips like a bubble of hope.

"That's right!" I laugh, delighted at his tiny voice echoing my thoughts.

Rhythmic Reverence

Love washes through me, erasing my pain—pain housed within me since my first breath. My son's eyelids flutter, the ache in my legs softens, and the pain loosens its grip. My body remembers how it feels to be loved.

Love is a sound, and I move with it through the rocking motion of the bentwood. The repetitive rhythms wrap our home in a sacred hush. I ache for enlightenment and yearn to learn. His stomach rises and falls in rhythmic renewal, and I attune to the cadence of his breath.

He kicks his feet, a soft *thump-thump* against my chest, and the rhythmic release begins.

"Okay," I say, brushing a tear from my cheek. "Let's do this." I sing and rock in reverence, entering an embodied presence of divine flow.

The soothing sound pulses through my veins, sparks cellular memories, settles into my bones, and awakens me to Source. It's not just a melody, but a transformational rhythmic journey, supported by generations of beings seeking spiritual reverence. It is kinship.

We rock and cuddle, wrapped in a cozy blanket of inexpressible joy. A familiar voice whispers to me in the hush of the night.

The sound is always with you. Just follow the rhythm in your heart.

The Ebb and Flow

Outside the window, the moon peeks out from beneath a dark blue cloud, illuminating the grass and evergreens with a magical glow. It casts soft shadows across my floor. I stop and start humming with each inhale and exhale.

Stop and start.
In and out.
Begin and end.

I breathe and sing in sync with a universal rhythm aligned with the breath and heartbeat of the world. The movement of the rocking chair matches the ebb and flow of my breath, and the intermittent silence is as sweet as the sound.

I move—not only forward and backward, but inward and outward to align with the music of the spheres.

Do you hear me, Jean?

Who are you?

I am always with you. The rhythm of your heart and breath is one with the sacred sound of the universe. It's the pulse within you. You are never alone.

A beating pulse stirs within me, coaxing original melodies and soothing words from the marrow of my being. As I sing a gentle lullaby to my son, I sing to myself—healing old wounds with melodies of comfort and care. Slowly, I recognize the unique pitch and timbre of the voice flowing through me. It is deeply familiar, stirring a longing ache in my heart— quiet, steady, and tender. I speak to the universe, asking for comfort and wisdom.

Is this why my pain softened?

Yes. You've been hating your pain, but love remembers you, because you remember love. Life's energies flow like the ebb and flow of the tide, but love is always here, and you know how to find it.

It is my mother's voice. Her melody moves through me with rhythmic reverence. Her cadence aligns with mine, echoing through generations of women who sang to survive, to soothe, to love—an ancient lineage of those who clapped, rocked, wrote, moved, and sang through life's challenges.

I place my son's head on my shoulder, near my heart, with my palm holding his neck and back. I stand and gently swirl around the room, dancing to the rhythm of life. I radically change my perspective.

I lose my desire to fix my life, or others in it. I shift—gently, deliberately—to embrace my responsibility for disciplined self-care. With each breath, I begin the daily practice of healing from a lifetime of chronic pain.

Embodied Rhythm

It's late morning in the sunlit therapy room. I sit on the edge of a padded table, my legs weighted heavily with armor. My physical therapist, Lena, sits beside me with a clipboard in hand.

"Hello. You made it. That's a win. How are you feeling today, Jean?"

"I'm great, but the vestibular migraine hit me before I got out of bed this morning. I'm still coming out of it, so pardon my drunken speech."

Lena motions for me to stand up. "Today is our eval day." She winks with a chipper smile, coaxing me to embrace the pain. "I'll follow you."

"Okay. Let's go!" I say with gumption and grace.

I struggle as I walk with my cane, braced legs dragging across the carpeted hallway. We pass the reception area, decked out in festive Halloween decorations—skeletons grinning, pumpkins glowing. I can't help but laugh at my robotic steps.

"I walk like Frankenstein's monster, tramping through the fog with 300-pound weights on my ankles."

Lena chuckles beside me. It feels good to be with someone who appreciates the humor of pain.

"More like 500-pound weights, not 300. Are you hurting? Should we stop? Maybe you should bring your walker or wheelchair next time."

I shake my head.

"No, I've been walking like this for a lifetime. I couldn't be happier unless there were two of me," I say, offering a small laugh and smile.

Lena encourages me. "Muscle fatigue is common with migraines and mechanical injuries. You're doing fine."

I silently chant my gratitude mantra.

Left foot—*Grate.*
Right foot—*ful.*
Left foot—*Grate.*
Right foot—*ful.*

The syllables echo through my body, each one with a soft drumbeat of resilience and grace. My heart opens to the quiet blessings of breath, motion, and presence, as I ride the waves.

Pain is here, but I only feel joy.

THE WELLNESS WARRIORS

Lena walks behind me with a counting device, tracking each step to record my progress. We pass framed scenic paintings by local artists—wild brushstrokes, waves crashing in rhythmic surrender. I imagine the artist's hand moving like mine: slow, deliberate, and alive. Six minutes later, we arrive back at the starting point.

"Nailed it." I laugh.

Ebb and flow. Ebb and flow.

"Okay. Let's sit for a minute." She guides me through repetitive arm movements, measuring flexion, and extension.

"Hey, your range of motion is up from last month. That's good." Her perky ponytail bobs as she quickly turns her head, opens the drawer, and returns the goniometer and inclinometer to their rightful homes.

"I'm limitless!"

Lena winks at me and turns to type something on the computer, staring at the monitor while chatting. "Keep doing the vestibular resets and ankle stretches daily, even if just for a few minutes. One breath, one step, one goal. Pause, breathe, listen to your body, and stop if it hurts."

The rattling noise of the printer breaks the silence as Lena reaches forward to hand me a paper with photographic illustrations—my assignment for the week.

"Thanks so much for your patience. You're my cheerleader." I collect my jacket and purse while she rises from the chair.

"Well, thank *you* for being patient too. Some days you will hurt, and it will feel slow. Other days will be faster. Look around. You're not alone."

There it was again. I am not alone.

I pause, scanning the room and seeing others like me—brave wellness warriors who embrace pain to shift and uplift themselves and others. They're dancing to the rhythm of life, going with the ebb and flow. This is my community, my inspiration, and motivation.

This cadence is always here, whether a sound is heard, limbs move, or eyes see. I discover rhythmic reverence when I look, listen, and move with an ethereal beat found in all living things. It is always with me and always with you.

Removing the Cloak

As I leave the physical therapist, I feel grateful, joyful, and alive. Yet, gripping emotional and physical pain is always with me. As a child, teen, and adult, I struggled with managing this dark cloak around my heart: a shadow of shame associated with chronic pain and illness.

My mother was uncomfortable with emotions, yet I love and understand her now.

"You're so sensitive and dramatic. What's the matter? Stop crying."

"I can't help it. I'm sad."

"What have you got to be sad about?"

That question isn't easily answered—not by anyone living with chronic pain. Most people wrongly believe that depression needs a reason: a lost job, a broken heart, a shattered bone, a house in flames. But that's a myth. Depression and suicidal ideation often rise from invisible roots: silent injuries, unseen grief, neurological storms.

A quiet voice inside me accompanies my pain.

I want to die.
I want to chop off my arms and legs.
I want to chop off my head.

I've lived with chronic depression most of my life, shaped by multiple concussions and mechanical injuries beginning at age three. Depression is not a failure. It's a companion—a normal response to a body that's been navigating pain for decades.

And yet, I experience joy every day, beyond my wildest imagination. Perhaps even more than the average Joe. People tell me daily that I light up the room with joy. So how do I do it?

I embrace both chronic pain and chronic joy.
I move through life with rhythmic renewal and reverence.
I do it. And you can too.

REBUILDING RHYTHM AND BEATING PAIN

After more than seventy years in this body, I still experience daily thoughts of suicide—not with intent, but as a quiet undertow. Passive suicidal ideation isn't a crashing wave. It's not a plan or a decision. It's a soft pull beneath the surface of daily life. It doesn't kick and scream. It whispers. Invisible to others, it moves with me in every breath. A quiet weeping bathes my heart, yet I consciously choose gratitude and joy. I laugh, love, and live my life in joyful celebration.

The hawk circles overhead, its cry slicing through the morning hush. I treasure our nature walks with Pumpkin, my husband, and our matching canes.

My deaf husband signs to me, his silver hair shining in the sun, "That bird walks better than we do."

I laugh, signing back, "And it hears better, too."

He grins. "Speak for yourself. I'm still handsome." We both chuckle; our rhythm is slow but steady, stitched together by humor and love.

For those living with chronic pain or neurological injury, the undertow is familiar. Not feared—navigated. Chronic pain increases the risk of depression, anxiety, and suicide. A 2023 twin study of over 17,000 people found a 51% greater risk of suicidal behavior in those with high levels of chronic pain. I accept pain as a companion, a reminder of the strength I summon each day.

Here's the amazing grace: rhythm heals.

Research shows that rhythmic activity improves depression, anxiety, memory, and emotional regulation. All are vital in trauma recovery. Drumming lowers cortisol, boosts immunity, and rewires the brain. The rhythmic rhyme of poetry helps reframe pain and reclaim feelings, power, and intention. Dance offers somatic release and emotional freedom.

My husband and I pause beneath a tree, watching the hawk glide. I imagine the undertow beneath its wings—unseen, but powerful. That's what it feels like. The hawk flies near us, tipping its wing as it passes over our heads.

"I love my life."

"Me, too."

I'm proud of my life, my husband, and our disabilities. I'm grateful for the joy and pain. I'm not alone, and neither are you.

I survive by leaning into rhythm. My training as a music therapist and expressive arts teacher gives me what I need—daily tools—not just for others, but for myself. Embodied rhythm helps me move, connect, and rise in a drug-free, safe, and easy manner.

Each step is a drumbeat of belonging. Each sway is a sacred sound, memory, and rhythm that heals when other treatments fail.

From Ache to Awake

I linger in the dream world—weightless, warm, and cradled in divine love. Pain doesn't follow me, light doesn't hurt me, and harsh sounds don't rattle my brain. Soft sounds soothe me with the swish of angel wings and hum of the galaxies.

But the veil thins. It's time to wake up.

Returning to my physical body is like slipping into a garment that no longer fits. The ache is waiting—familiar, pulsing, patient. My lids resist. The pillow is cool and soft. I breathe.

A sliver of light slices in. White. Sharp. Blinding. I flinch. Then soften.

"Good morning, Pain," I whisper. "I love you. It's another beautiful day. Let's go."

We are not alone. We're connected by the cadence of our hearts, the movement of the blood dancing through our veins, and the poetic sound of our words, connecting to those who walked before us and those with us today.

We are a community, living within a circle of sound and light and moving to it and through it in reverent renewal. Rhythmic restoration is safe, effective, and easy. Why not try it now? Below are the tools I use daily to shift and uplift from pain to joy.

THE TOOL

Rhythm is found in all life—the breath, the heartbeat, and all the body systems, the spinning of the planets, the rising and setting of the sun, birth, death, and the four seasons. Life depends on rhythm and cannot survive without it.

When we feel out of sync, we must align ourselves with the natural rhythm of life: tune in, tune out, and tune up. We do this through rhythmic restoration, renewal, and reverence. The expressive arts are powerful tools for achieving balance through creative modalities such as drumming, chanting, movement, painting, and poetry. Rhythm helps us release emotions and express ourselves through creative flow.

MODALITIES

You can choose from any number of materials or keep it simple with a blank piece of paper, pen, or pencil. Have your supplies ready before beginning.

1. Visual Art – paper, pen, paint, clay, collage, needlework, craft supplies

2. Photography – camera, natural light, meaningful objects

3. Music – instruments, voice, clapping, tapping, recorded sound

4. Dance – safe space, music, scarves, breath-led movement

5. Drama – props, costumes, scripts, improvisation

6. Gardening – soil, seeds, pots, tools, water

7. Cooking – ingredients, utensils, rhythm in stirring and chopping

8. Creative Writing – paper, pen, laptop, recording device

9. Textile Arts – weaving, quilting, embroidery, knitting, braiding

10. Nature Rituals – walking, stone stacking, leaf arranging

DAILY PRACTICE

Where do you experience rhythm? Begin making a list. Schedule time on your calendar every day if possible, or several times a week.

1. Morning chant or prayer

2. Writing rhythmic poems or affirmations

3. Rocking to regulate breath

4. Drumming or tapping feet/fingers throughout the day

5. Playing a musical instrument

6. Singing a song or humming a tune

7. Dancing around the room

8. Running or walking in nature

9. Planting flowers or tending a garden

10. Folding clothes with intention

11. Washing dishes mindfully

12. Stirring soup, scrambling an egg, or whipping cream

13. Bathing, or washing, curling, or braiding hair

14. Listening to birdsong or ocean waves

15. Sweeping, dusting, or mopping the floor

EXPLORE YOUR OWN RHYTHM

1. Sit quietly. Feel your pain. Feel your joy. Introduce them to one another.

2. Breathe deeply, exhale sound, practice saying words, find your word.

3. Move. Choose your way of moving: tap, chant, sway, write, dance, etc.

4. Listen to the heart beating within you. Thank your heart. Receive its gift.

5. Feel your pulse, let the rhythm of your pulse guide you deeply to your heart.

6. Notice the rhythm of your breath: fast, slow, shallow, deep, etc.

7. Name your rhythm. Thank it for its uniqueness.

8. Mirror your rhythm. Echo it with movement or sound.

9. Express your rhythm outwardly: clap, hum, journal, speak, dance.

10. Rest in reverence. Thank your body. Thank your rhythm. Thank your pain.

Remember: You are not your pain. You are rhythm, breath, and light. Your unique rhythm carries you home. When we walk with chronic pain and not against it, rhythm is the path, renewal is the doorway, and reverence is the key. If you are suffering and looking for simple, safe, soothing methods to manage pain, visit my website for more information. You are not alone.

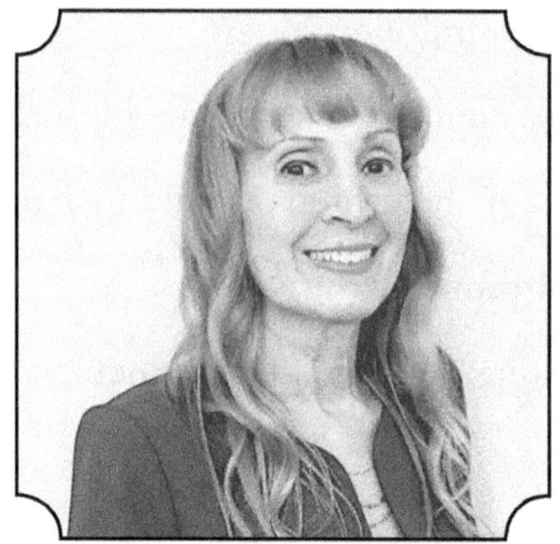

Jean Voice Dart, MS, RMT, is a multiple international best-selling author, expressive arts psychotherapist, coach, and teacher who navigated through grief, trauma, and chronic pain, upleveling her life from stressed to blessed. She has witnessed a lifetime of miraculous transformations, helping others feel, reveal, and heal through the arts. Those working with Jean spark creative flow, fine-tune skills, and gain effective strategies to manage life challenges through the expressive arts (art, music, writing, movement, and drama). She currently lives near the Pacific Ocean, with her husband, Matt, and their dog, Pumpkin.

CREDENTIALS

- Certified Expressive Arts Grief and Trauma Coach (CCF)

- Certified Art Therapy Practitioner (CATP)

- Credentialed adult continuing education teacher (music, fine arts, creative writing)

- Credentialed Teacher K-12 (MS, in Special Education)

- Group and private music, art, theater, and writing teacher, primary and secondary

- Registered Music Therapist (RMT)

- More than fifty years of experience as a therapist, teacher, performer, presenter, coach, and speaker

REFERENCES

Nahin, Richard L. "Estimates of Pain Prevalence and Impact Among Adults in the United States, 2023." National Center for Health Statistics, U.S. Department of Health and Human Services, 2024.

Bittman, Barry B., et al. "Composite Effects of Group Drumming Music Therapy on Modulation of Neuroendocrine-Immune Parameters in Normal Subjects." *Alternative Therapies in Health and Medicine* 7, no. 1 (2001): 38–47.

Fancourt, Daisy, and Saoirse Finn. "What Is the Evidence on the Role of the Arts in Improving Health and Well-Being?" World Health Organization, 2019.

Thaut, Michael H. *Rhythm, Music, and the Brain: Scientific Foundations and Clinical Applications.* New York: Routledge, 2005.

Winkelman, Michael. "Shamanism and Cognitive Evolution." *Cambridge Archaeological Journal* 20, no. 1 (2010): 75–94.

CONNECT WITH JEAN:

Website: https://www.jeanvoicedart.com

Contact: https://www.jeanvoicedart.com/contact

Facebook: https://www.facebook.com/jeanvoicedartauthor

Instagram: https://www.instagram.com/jeanvoicedart

LinkedIn: https://www.linkedin.com/in/jeanvoicedart

Pain can become background noise, part of the 'normal' you manage instead of question.

~ Sandra Lee

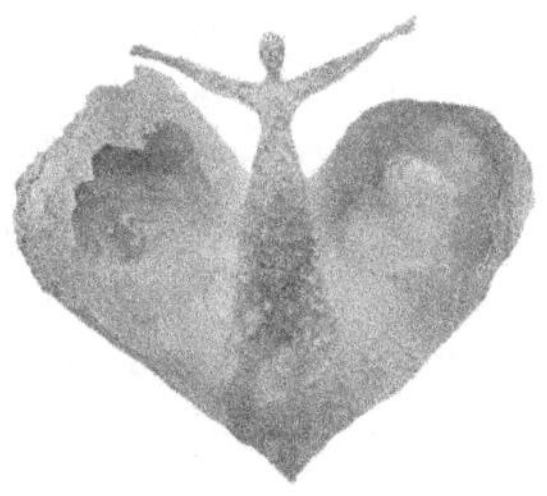

Stories Become Symptoms, Stories Heal
Breathe Beyond Pain for Freedom

Sandra Lee

BS, LMT

I can't do this alone.

That thought beat differently in my heart than it ever had before, its voice a soft whisper instead of a shout. Like flipping a switch, the dark room lit up, and the pain began to melt.

For years, that belief filled my head and stopped my hands. Then, in a flash of healing and release, the comfortable certainty of *I can't do this* dissolved away.

Have you ever reached a breaking point—resisted as long and hard as you could, then, in an explosion of awareness, released a familiar yet restrictive handhold and discovered a clarity that had been there all along? "Why didn't I see this before?"

You couldn't see it until it was your time.

MY STORY

For years, I tore my hair out struggling to build success on my own, the perfectly aligned business I felt in my bones.

Entrepreneurship is fucking hard work! Unfortunately, nobody explains this until you're already buried way over your head.

My business provided an endless cycle of opportunities to hesitate and distract myself. And the familiar sitcom rerun, "I Can't Do This Alone," played on repeat.

Each time I felt lost about how to tackle the next business step, I froze and wanted to quit. This fed suicidal thoughts. When I bit my lip, determined to push through to complete some task, another impossible-feeling action was always sitting on my tail, waiting next in line.

Then came the month I couldn't pay the credit card bill. I freaked out. In desperation, I grabbed for programs the flashy experts promised were just the right solution.

Valiantly, I jumped in and promised myself: *I can do it,* only to run face-first into the wall of the two super-basic questions that pushed me into panicked confusion every time.

"Who do you serve? And what's the benefit you provide for them?"

The fancy programs didn't deliver solutions for me. They upped the ante on my endless *I can't do this* hamster wheel race. And the only destination I reached was deeper debt.

In my heart, I knew all the barriers were in my mind, yet I couldn't identify the way through.

The pressure of continual stress on my body felt like an ever-familiar bracing throughout my solar plexus, shoulders, and arms. And yes, sometimes it was excruciatingly painful. I was just deaf to the message.

When I slowed down enough to notice, I realized my entire right side was guarding, held, coiled like a snake waiting to protect against an attack that never came.

An emotionally sensitive practitioner asked, "What is held in there?" Immediately, the answer called out: *Everything I haven't allowed myself to do.*

This was a prelude for what was to come.

HEALING

The eleven intensive days of my Neurolinguistic Programming (NLP) master certification training provided a crucible, heating and concentrating my issues so I could experience a transformative breakthrough session.

In NLP, a breakthrough is a series of coach-guided processes that provide healing for limiting decisions, unresolved emotions, and the root stories that drive unhelpful patterns.

This was it—my opportunity to heal, *'I can't do this'* at the roots, and to release the ineffectiveness that plagued me for decades.

When I was six months old, my parents left me with an aunt and an uncle for three days. To an infant, three days is forever. I freaked, screamed my lungs out, and frantically tried everything imaginable. My body was certain: *Mother's not coming back. I'm on my own.*

Without words or logic, I made other decisions too, decisions that shaped the rest of my life. The panicked *I can't do this alone* vows of an infant became unconscious rules for myself as an adult attempting to be an entrepreneur. I'm responsible for everything and everyone. If I don't do it, it won't get done. If I can't do it perfectly, I shouldn't even try.

It was breakthrough time in NLP, and I was deep into the process. All of my ineffectiveness and struggles from the past came to the show. My throat tightened; tears flowed everywhere. My neck and head ached the same way they always did when I pushed myself.

My coach prompted, "See your mother in front of you. What do you need to hear from her?" The dam burst, and out of my sobbing heart flowed wave after wave of words I'd swallowed my entire life.

After what seemed like forever, the flow moment of transition came. Time stood still, and colors sharpened. I saw the soft lamplight on the desk and felt the tear-soaked handkerchief in my hand. The Earth's energy rose up through the chair, supporting me as I spoke.

"I am completely alone." That final wave crested, then released. And I sobbed until the charge was depleted. My exhausted crying eased, and a quiet settled inside me.

And the pain in my neck? The pain that chiropractors, massage therapists, and energy healers poked at for years? It let go.

That was the crux. I exhaled a slow, audible sigh, and a heavy curtain lifted.

The keystone pattern anchoring my physical pain wasn't actually in the muscles; it was a belief formed before I had words. And that belief drove my business, relationships, body—everything.

Before this release, I told my coach, "I need proof that these old patterns can be let go of. The evidence I want is the pain in my neck going away."

SOURCE AND ABUNDANCE

Intellectually, I believed in God or Source, because I saw how life appeared to flow for other people. Clients called, opportunities unfolded, and unexpected inheritances appeared. But Source certainly couldn't be there for me.

During the breakthrough, the puzzle pieces fell into place, and my most profound realization landed. As we concluded the breakthrough process, I spoke it out loud: "I'm alone. Source is not here for me." There was no divine safety net.

I had never seen this particular facet of my helplessness before. Saying it felt like admitting a private truth I built a life around.

When the wave of release came and the pain eased, it was a miracle. There was no logic to it. My body provided the proof that Source is here for me. I am not alone.

This experience didn't just restore my faith in Source; it renewed my confidence as a healer. I knew, in my own tissues, that when people reach the root decision underlying their symptoms, change can be immediate and material.

Since then, I've guided clients to find freedom from pain by uncovering the old decisions within their patterns and releasing them.

What This Means for You

If you live with pain, the Tool below is for you. It helps you understand what your body is trying to say through pain and tension, guiding your awareness toward the deeper issues beneath your symptoms. As you begin to heal those underlying patterns, even long-term pain can ease, and real, lasting relief becomes possible.

If you have pain that whispers while you work, tension on the right side, or a neck that tightens whenever you step toward visibility, I see you. If you're brilliant and capable yet still find yourself signing up for programs and stalling, I've been there.

You may be juggling clients, family, and aging parents, carrying more than anyone realizes. Your body absorbs the pressure to keep everyone happy. The strain of pushing forward, doing what must be done, settles into tight shoulders, an aching head, or a weary lower back.

Pain can become background noise, part of the 'normal' you manage rather than question. Choosing to heal means drawing pain back into the light. Its depths may reveal decisions your body made long ago about safety, responsibility, visibility, or worth. When you consciously reframe those decisions, your body's holding begins to soften, and pain shifts when your system feels safe again.

The Tool helps you begin cracking open old experiences and reconsidering long-assumed truths. Have easeful conversations with your nervous system, organizing your experiences into a structure: evidence of success, clarity about patterns, and small, doable next steps. Create something you can see on paper, say out loud, and feel in your body.

This process also opens a doorway into your unconscious mind, the vault of your hidden stories. The unconscious holds everything you've ever experienced, including turning point moments when your system decided what was safe or unsafe.

Imagine each bit of unresolved experience as an energy bubble stored by your unconscious. When the bubbles formed, it wasn't safe or possible for your conscious mind to process them, so your system tucked them away.

As you heal, the bubbles resurface as whispers calling out, "Pay attention! Healing is available." They may appear as stabs of pain when you ask for help, arguments with your children, or projects that keep stalling. Recognizing these as signals for awareness, rather than problems, opens the door to new choices that bring ease, freedom, and trust in your body's ability to heal.

Sometimes the whispers lead deeper than you can go alone. Working with a skilled practitioner can help you move through them safely and effectively.

That's how it was for me. My whispers were pain, overwhelm, and a business that was going nowhere. On my own, I was too close to myself to recognize that I believed Source was not there for me. Recognizing and naming that truth transformed it. I knew the barriers were in my mind, yet I couldn't do it alone. When I was ready, my tearful breakthrough was massive, and everything shifted.

Before we dive into The Tool, here's a quick note on safety and scope. This chapter shares my personal experience and a tool for self-inquiry. It's for day-to-day challenges. If you have or suspect a medical or mental health condition, consult a licensed professional. If distress or trauma memories arise, pause, ground yourself, and reach out for support.

THE TOOL

Before you begin, put a *Do Not Disturb* sign on the door and turn on relaxing music. Grab a notebook and pen (or open a document), pour a glass of water or a cup of tea, and settle into a comfortable chair. Set your journal beside you for insights. Take a sip, slow your breathing, and let your soft-eyed gaze settle on a calming point across the room. Take a deep breath and exhale any tension.

Select the questions below that provide clarity and reveal insights.

If difficulties arise, see "Troubleshooting" at the end of the tool.

STEP 1: A WIN AND A CHALLENGE

- **Your Win.** Choose an area of your life or business where you feel accomplished.

  - Describe why this matters to you.

  - What is happening? What do you see yourself doing?

  - What are your thoughts about it?

  - What does it look like, sound like, and feel like?

  - What do you notice in your body?

  - Optional question. Do you feel connected to, or guided by Source in this area?

- **Your Challenge.** Choose an area that is not the way you would like it to be. Select a Challenge that is meaningful but manageable. Do not choose a major trauma.

  - Describe why this matters to you.

  - Describe what is happening and how it impacts you.

  - What do you see yourself doing?

  - What are your thoughts?

  - What does it look like, sound like, and feel like?

  - What do you notice in your body?

  - Optional question. Do you feel connected to, or guided by Source in this area?

Examples:

- **My Win:** As a massage therapist, I love helping people feel and function better. I love it when they stand up from the massage table, surprised to find the pain in their shoulder is gone, and they walk better.

- **Challenge:** I really struggled with making phone calls (I used to). When I needed to make them, I felt overwhelmed and had knots in my gut. I used to escape to the kitchen and scour the refrigerator for food.

STEP 2: INSIGHTS

As you sit with your Win and your Challenge, you may see flashes of insight.

- Keep your journal handy and jot awarenesses down.

- Don't analyze yet. Just notice feelings, images, words, and sounds.

- Notice sensations and any pain or discomfort. For example: "My shoulders always tighten the day before a launch," or "I keep telling myself I'll figure it out alone."

STEP 3: CELEBRATE

- Name your Win out loud, and say why it matters.

- Let yourself feel what this represents.

- Place a hand on your heart or shoulders and say, "Good job."

- Do a happy dance.

This is not fluff. Your nervous system learns from celebration. When you acknowledge wins, your body registers safety in moving forward.

STEP 4: LOOK, LISTEN, AND FEEL

- Notice what you see and hear about your Challenge.

- Listen for the *voice* that pipes up.

- Write down the exact phrases you hear in your head.

- Note the tone and whether it sounds like anyone you know.

- Are there physical sensations (tight jaw, shallow breath, right shoulder grabbing)?

- You are mapping the links between thoughts, feelings, and body.

Examples of thoughts:

- *If I can't do it perfectly, why bother?*

- *I should already know how to do this.*

- *No one is coming to help me.*

- *It's safer not to be visible.*

- *I always quit anyway.*

STEP 5: COMPARE AND CHOOSE

- Notice how differently you experience your Win and your Challenge.

- Record any realizations.

- Are there actions you feel drawn to take?

STEP 6: TINY ACTION WITHIN 24 HOURS

- Choose one micro action related to your Challenge: draft one sentence of a call script, send a text to schedule a call, or leave yourself a 30-second practice voicemail.

- Keep it under five minutes so success feels easy.

STEP 7: CARRY YOUR INSIGHTS INTO THE PAIN AWARENESS QUIZ

- The Pain Awareness Quiz helps you hear the messages your pain is trying to send you. Take a few minutes to complete it, free.

  Here is the link: https://shinewithsandra.com/quiz

TROUBLESHOOTING

- **If no Win comes to mind:** look back over your last week and pick any moment you felt even a little proud or relieved. Anything that turned up the corners of your mouth or opened your heart counts.

- **If the Challenge feels too big:** choose a smaller slice, something you can positively influence this week.

- **If you're tapping into a major trauma:** pause. Skip the big issues now and work with a qualified professional.

- **If tears or numbness show up:** pause and be gentle with yourself. You're touching upon meaningful memories. Return to the present moment. Breathe, look around, and name three objects you see, two sounds you hear, and one emotion or sensation you feel. Sip water and return to this memory later.

- **If the inner critic gets loud:** write its exact words, then ask, "What is this voice trying to protect me from?" Thank it and continue.

CASE STUDY

Bethany (not her real name) is a coach in her fifties. When we met, she had had a headache every day for thirteen months. Each morning, the one thing she knew for certain was, "I will have a headache today." It drained her energy, attention, and hope. She saw multiple doctors, completed sleep studies, and took expensive medication, yet the pain continued.

After our first session, her headache lifted, followed by three full days without pain. The headaches did return, but the break gave her something she hadn't felt in a while: evidence that a future without headaches was possible. We began Neurolinguistic Programming (NLP) to reveal the roots of the pain, including the stored stress patterns her body was carrying and the stories that triggered them. Over time, the headaches became less frequent and less intense, and she learned to notice early signs and settle her system.

She became excited about sharing her creative work, and a potential romantic partner entered her life. Most importantly, she began to feel like herself; she could meet people, enjoy time with them, and build the life she wanted.

Your Next Step: Take the Pain Awareness Quiz

If you are curious about your own pain patterns, take the **Pain Awareness Quiz,** my gift to you. Access the free quiz here: https://shinewithsandra.com/quiz

Take a few minutes for this short, eye-opening quiz to:

- See how your pain impacts your emotions, self-care, and sense of control.

- Understand the hidden messages your body is sending.

- Identify where you are on the path to freedom from pain.

- Discover your next steps toward increased energy, clarity, and ease.

  Your body is speaking. This quiz helps you hear what it's really saying.

You will also receive a short series of supportive emails with simple tips you can use immediately.

When You Are Ready For Deeper Change

If this chapter resonated, and you would appreciate support in uncovering and releasing the decisions underlying your pain, I'd love to talk. In a private conversation, we can explore options and create a path toward ease, momentum, and freedom. See the bio for contact information and to book a **Freedom from Pain Action Plan Call.**

Closing

My breakthrough began with a sentence I didn't know was shaping my life.

What is the key to your liberation?

Your successes tell a story of resilience. Your challenges point toward areas you're ready to turn around. When you meet those places with compassion, clarity, and support from trusted people, from your inner wisdom, and from Source, your body can step forward to meet you with relief.

In your life filled with real responsibilities, small, consistent steps matter. Pace yourself and open the door to support. That's how we heal: one step at a time until the path looks clearer, your voice sounds steadier, and your body feels safer.

Breathe

Love, *Gandra Lee*

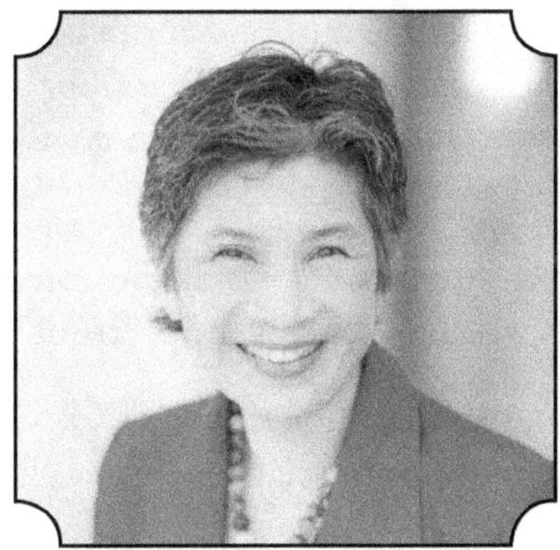

Sandra Lee, BS, LMT, is the owner of Miracle Inspirations and a mentor who has helped hundreds of women entrepreneurs stop pushing through pain and start living fully with clarity and confidence. She specializes in migraine and headache relief. Clients describe her results as "miraculous."

With over 30 years in massage, intuitive, energetic, and sound healing, and a Caltech BS in chemistry, she blends science and energy to help clients visualize the 'science' of their bodies and release patterns holding pain in place. Speak to the real root of symptoms, and the body changes.

Sandra is a Neurolinguistic Programming (NLP) Certified Master Practitioner, Biofield Tuning Practitioner, and Human Design Specialist.

What's next? I suggest these steps:

- **Pain Awareness Quiz:** gain insight into how pain impacts your freedom to be, and what to do next.
  Link: https://shinewithsandra.com/quiz

- **Freedom from Pain Action Plan Call:** a conversation to map your next steps to liberation from symptoms.
  Link: https://shinewithsandra.com/cc

- **Bonus. Ground & Release Stress:** energetically reset with a short Biofield Tuning audio.
  Link: https://shinewithsandra.com/bookresources

A healer, speaker, and best-selling author, Sandra contributed to *The Energy Medicine Solution: Mind Blowing Results for Living an Extraordinary Life,* and to two books about Human Design, *Stop Overworking and Start Overflowing* and *Abundance By Design.*

Creator of **The Anger Spectrum**™ and the **Breathe Beyond Pain**™ **Framework,** Sandra is writing The Anger Spectrum™ book.

Living with her husband in British Columbia's Okanagan Valley, Canada, she also visits Washington State to see friends and clients.

CONNECT WITH SANDRA:

LinkedIn: https://www.linkedin.com/in/sandra-lee-701662250

Facebook: https://www.facebook.com/SandraLeeInspiration

Instagram: https://www.instagram.com/miracleinspirations

YouTube: https://www.youtube.com/@sandralee1miracleinspirations

Empowering you to find freedom from pain.

Breathe

Sandra Lee

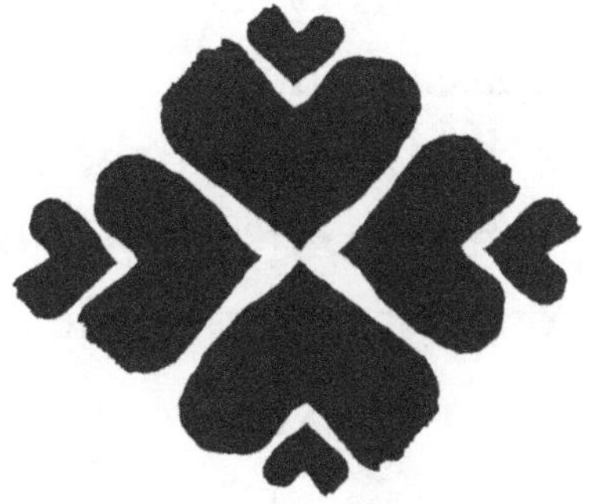

Healing through this type of deception taught me that compassion doesn't mean assuming someone else's discomfort at the expense of my own peace or health. It means holding both empathy and self-respect in the same breath and space.

~ Donna O'Toole

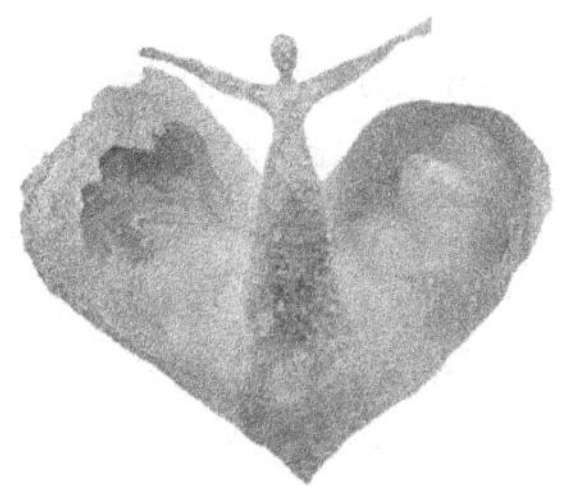

CHAPTER 11

LIES OF OMISSION
RISING FROM THE SILENCE OF BETRAYAL TO BECOMING ME

Donna O'Toole

R.N., REIKI MASTER, END OF LIFE DOULA

MY STORY

Unspoken truths have a way of echoing until you can no longer ignore them. I learned silence wounds more deeply than the truth ever could. As I sat in the painful silence of his betrayal, I surprisingly discovered the many ways I had silenced myself. Rising from the pain and deep wounds of deception required courage to reclaim my voice, truth, and trust. I arose from the ashes as a phoenix to become me.

Lies of Omission

What question should I be asking
That I do not know to ask?
And in that single question
Will I uncover your
Lies of Omission.

It was not the chosen words you spoke
But the words you selected

Not to be uttered from your lips
That slithered like a serpent up my body
And coiled its way around my tender heart.

When Lies of Omission are discovered,
The next questions become
What other Lies of Omission
Has he not spoken
And when was his
First Lie of Omission?
Doubt and Deception
Creep up my body
Winding their way
Adjoining the serpent
Around my tender heart.

When did you first start
To tell me the chosen story
You wanted me to believe?
I want to believe in my heart
You feel you did not lie to me.
But you just chose to tell
A version of your story
To leave out the parts
That would cause me to ask you questions
You never wanted to answer.
Perhaps, not to hurt me or
Was it so you always got what you wanted?

So, I sit with the apparitions
of your missing words,
Making up fictitious stories in my
wild and vivid imagination.
I wonder which versions of you
Are the man I think I know
Or are all these stories the
Dark shadow of the truths
Climbing the stairs
Striking the midnight clock
Of disillusion?

Will dawn awaken
The truths to be seen?
Can love survive
The woven webs of deceit?
Can you tell me
Not what I already know
But what I do not know
What you feel if you said
Would destroy what we have,
The love I hold for you.

Once you began to
Weave the webs of Omission
Know it is not your stories that
Cause me more hurt.
But it is the choices you made
That left me in the dark
And took away my power
To make my own decisions.

What question should I be asking
That I do not know to ask?

When David entered the room, I asked him, "Who is Ginger?"

"Why do you ask?" he replied.

With my heart pounding loudly in my throat, I somehow found enough voice to whisper, "Because she just posted a photo of the two of you on Facebook saying, 'When your boyfriend takes you out to dinner for your birthday.'"

I couldn't read the emotion on his face as David adamantly replied, "She is not my girlfriend. She's someone I used to date. We're just friends, and we have had an on-again-off-again relationship."

With further discussion, I learned he saw her often; they had common friends. Ginger lived close to David, and I lived three hours away. I understand that scenario.

"I am trying to figure out Ginger's and my relationship."

What did you just say? I could not have heard that right.

Stunned silence filled the room, but the words roaring inside my head were earth-shattering!

When did their relationship start? How often does he see her? How does he define friendship? Does he tell her we are just friends? Why is he with her? How intimate is he with her? What signs have I been missing? What signs have I chosen not to see?

My heart raced in beat with my thoughts.

I sat in disbelief as hurt began to rise in my heart and eyes. I don my mask of not letting anyone see my emotions. I'm good at this self-defensive move; I've used it for 65 years.

And then he just had to say, "Ginger wants to be with me for all the wrong reasons! She lives with her father."

"Stop. I don't want to hear anymore about her!"

Why does he think I want to know anything about her? I just want him to tell me that he loves me, and he is sorry he was seeing Ginger, and he will stop seeing her.

One half of my heart cried out for him to hold me. The other half wanted to bolt from the room. But I couldn't move, I was frozen in time, silenced by fear, not wanting to know, and wanting to know. Confusion clouded my thoughts until I remembered his declarations of love.

He loves me! I know he loves me!

"David, I believe the unique love we have for each other can weather this situation. I know you love me, and I know you understand the depth of love I hold for you. I will support you as you make this decision, as I know the love and connection we have together." "Thank you," he replied.

Our intense love and passion were overwhelming for him. David chose the easier path, one in which he settled or believed he could not be the person I saw him as being, his true essence. Sometimes people choose not to be the best version of themselves.

Two months later, he ghosted me. This pain was far worse than the lies of omission. Not having personal closure or understanding of his decisions almost destroyed me. His last words to me were, "We need to talk." And instead, I got silence, the deafening silence.

Seriously?! I never thought he'd be a coward to face me and tell me the truth. Or is he afraid of his feelings if he sees me?

There's a cost when you don't set certain boundaries in a relationship. Looking back, there were red flags. I saw them—gently waving at first, then flailing in the wind.

And what did I do? Of course, I chose to look away and bury my head in the sand. I told myself that unconditional love meant providing space and time for the relationship to unfold on its own, accepting everything, even the silence. I thought love required endless patience, that if I waited long enough, he'd eventually speak all his truths.

But love without boundaries is not unconditional love. This type of love is unsustainable. As I tried to understand his distance, I neglected my own pain. As I allowed space for his story, I suppressed my own voice.

I was teaching him that my needs did not matter as much as his—and even worse, I taught myself the same thing.

When I ignored the red flags, it was not because I was foolish, desperate, or lacked intelligence. It was because I loved David deeply and wanted to believe the best in him, even when he was not ready to meet me in the same way. But real love does not thrive in avoidance. It grows in truth. And truth requires courage—the courage to speak, set boundaries, and say "this hurts me" before the silence hardens into distance, and then no more communication.

Healing through this type of deception taught me that compassion doesn't mean assuming someone else's discomfort at the expense of my own peace or health. It means holding both empathy and self-respect in the same breath and space.

I learned that unconditional love should never mean unconditional self-sacrifice.

It means loving with an open heart while setting mutually healthy boundaries.

I certainly believe that if two people love each other and are willing to put in the time to earn each other's trust, then anything is possible.

Seven months later, I sat at the Riande Restaurant in Panama, where we had met two years earlier, and stared at the empty chair. I sat with so many emotions—hurt, disappointment, anger, disbelief, sorrow, love, distrust, joy, passion, friendship, laughter, sadness, connection, hope—allowing them to flow through me. *I know I still need time for my heart to heal.*

I continue to gaze at the chair that held so much connection and hope with this man. A few tears quietly spill over from the corner of my right eye and gently flow down my face to land on my napkin.

I'm grateful to have discovered an amazing love in my 70s and know I'm worthy of so much more.

When Clarity Comes Knocking

It is not just in any one moment,
But an accumulation of many things,
When clarity seems to
Come out of nowhere,
Appearing suddenly and
Unexpectedly welcomed.

Understanding that
Love is not enough
When it has nowhere to go.

There were no fanfares,
No warnings,
But in the presence of
Only one heartbeat
I am aware

I can breathe easily
As I emerge from
My cocoon,
Freeing myself from the
Bondages of my past.

I am the butterfly,
and
I set myself free,
Shedding old patterns and
Embracing new beginnings.

Flapping my wings,
Getting my bearings
I yearn for flight.

I let go.
I let it go.
I let you go.

I am choosing
To rebirth myself
On my new journey.
Joyfully loving each and every day,
Listening to my voice within,
Awakening fresh ideas and
Rising to breathtaking heights.

I am free to fly
In any direction.
Wondering where the winds
Will entice me
To adventure today.

I reach to the heavens
Transversing the currents
Bravely soaring to unknown places,
Being authentic and
Becoming everything
I was meant to be.

Come soar with me.
Fly in Freedom,
Fly in joy, love, and light,
Fly with abandonment.

I am the butterfly,
Free to be Me.

THE TOOL

TRUTH AND CLARITY
HEALING AND INSIGHTFUL GUIDE

This guide unites two powerful healing journeys: the T.R.U.T.H. (Tell, Recognize, Understand, Transformation, Heal) and the C.L.A.R.I.T.Y. (Center, Listen, Accept, Reframe, Integrate, Trust, Yes). Together, they help one move from the silence and betrayal toward self-awareness, forgiveness, and personal empowerment.

THE T.R.U.T.H.: HEALING THE SILENCE

T—TELL YOURSELF THE TRUTH

Healing Insight: Naming the truth reclaims personal power and begins the process of freeing oneself from the story one has been telling oneself.

Stop the story you've told yourself to reclaim your voice. Naming the truth is the first act to heal your silence.

- What truth have I been avoiding about this situation?

- What truth have I been avoiding about myself?

- What emotions surface when I allow myself to acknowledge what happened?

- What story have I told myself to survive this pain?

- If I could speak freely, what would I say about what truly happened?

R—RECOGNIZE THE WOUND

Healing Insight: Recognition is not assigning blame or making a judgment; it's the courage to see what still needs compassion and self-care.

Discover how betrayal or silence has affected your sense of self.

- Where do I still feel hurt, angry, or unseen? Feel where these emotions may be stored in your body. Send those areas love and compassion.

- How has this experience changed how I view trust and/or vulnerability?

- What part of me became silent to stay safe or keep peace?

- In what ways have I minimized my pain to avoid feeling it fully?

U—UNDERSTAND THE PATTERN

Healing Insight: Understanding transforms guilt into awareness—it reveals the survival strategies that no longer serve you and that you can release.

Ask yourself these questions to discover the deeper roots of silence, avoidance, or fear of confrontation.

- When did I first learn to stay silent to avoid conflict?

- What beliefs or family patterns taught me that silence was safer than truth?

- How do I respond when others hide things from me?

- Have I internalized the idea that my truth will hurt people or cause rejection?

T—TRANSFORMATION THROUGH EXPRESSION AND LETTING GO

Healing Insight: Expression turns pain into personal power. Speaking your truth breaks the silence that the betrayal feeds on.

Release your pain through authentic, creative, and truthful expression.

- What do I need to express that I have been holding in?

- If I could write a letter I would never send, what would I say?

- How can I express my truth in a way that honors my healing—through writing, art, or conversation?

- What new story about myself am I ready to tell?

H—HEAL BY RECLAIMING SELF-TRUST

Healing Insight: Healing is not about what they did—it's about how you rebuild your relationship with yourself and others.

It is about moving from victimhood to self-empowerment.

- What does honesty with me look like now?

- What boundaries or values must I protect to stay aligned with my truth?

- How can I ensure I never silence myself again out of fear or love?

- What am I ready to forgive in myself to move forward freely?

PART 2 – THE C.L.A.R.I.T.Y.: LIVING THE TRUTH

C—CENTER YOURSELF IN STILLNESS

Healing Insight: Stillness creates space for clarity to enter. This allows your emotions to settle, so the truth becomes visible without distortion.

Connect to the Earth, grounding in your body, and be present in the stillness before assigning any meaning.

- Where do I feel confusion, and what happens when I pause and breathe there?

- What truths become clearer when I am quiet and not reacting?

- How does silence feel to you when you choose it and do not force it?

L—LISTEN WITHOUT DEFENSIVENESS OR JUDGMENT

Healing Insight: True listening is surrender. It transforms conversation into connection and makes reconciliation possible.

Listen inwardly and outwardly with openness, not fear.

- What is my heart saying beneath my thoughts?

- When others speak truth to me, do I listen or prepare to defend?

- What does it feel like to be heard—and to hear myself fully?

A—ACCEPT WHAT IS, WITHOUT ILLUSION

Healing Insight: Acceptance is not agreement; it's freedom. By seeing reality as it is, you stop fighting the past and start living in the now.

Release the urge to rewrite or rationalize reality.

- What parts of the truth do I still resist accepting?

- How do I protect myself from stories that no longer serve me?

- Can I hold both the pain of what happened and the peace of what is?

R—REFRAME THE MEANING

Healing Insight: Reframing does not erase the pain—it redeems it. It's how you reclaim authorship of your story.

Transform perspective from victimhood to growth.

- What did this experience teach me about my strength?

- How can I reinterpret my wound as an awakening?

- What new meaning can evolve from my silence and my truth?

I—INTEGRATE THE LESSON

Healing Insight: Integration is transformation in motion. You're no longer reacting to pain. You're responding from awareness.

Let the healing reshape your behavior, not just your thoughts.

- What does living my life in alignment with my truth look like now?

- How can I practice integrity in small, daily choices?

- What boundaries reflect my new self-respect?

T—TRUST THE PROCESS

Healing Insight: Trust bridges the gap between discovery and peace. You don't need all the answers to walk in truth.

Let go of urgency; recognize and understand that healing unfolds over time. Be kind and compassionate to yourself.

- Can I trust that clarity will deepen as I live authentically?

- What fears arise when I feel uncertain about my growth?

- What buttons are pushed when people think you should be over the betrayal by now?

- How can I stay faithful to the journey even when I cannot see the outcome?

Y—YES TO GRACE

Healing Insight: Saying yes or yielding isn't a weakness—it's surrendering to wholeness. Grace is clarity's final light—where forgiveness and wisdom meet at the Y.

Release control and be open to forgiveness, compassion, and the flow of life.

- What does grace mean to me after betrayal?

- Can I forgive myself for the times I stayed silent or believed less of myself?

- How do I let love, not fear, shape who I am becoming?

TRUTH TO CLARITY

Healing through truth leads to clarity, and clarity sustains healing. Together, these frameworks guide you to do inner work—from silence to a deep connection—through honesty, courage, and compassion. The more deeply you honor your truth, the clearer and freer you become, until you rise from the silence of betrayal to become the best version of yourself.

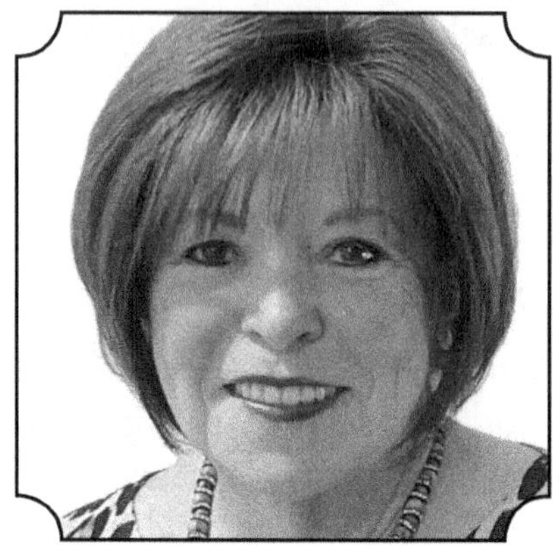

Donna O'Toole, RN, B.Ed., Intuitive, Energy Healer, End of Life Doula.

After caring for her husband of 14 years, who died from ALS, Donna knew something was missing from Western teachings. As a result, she studied and merged the Western and Eastern philosophies to enhance her healing abilities.

Donna is also a Reiki Master, a Karuna Reiki Master, and a crystal, sound, and color Healer. She's in her third decade of embracing the healing arts and energy work.

Donna's expertise focuses, as she feels called, on those individuals who need help with alternative healing options; transitioning from this earth plane; and those who have had the trauma of childhood sexual abuse.

Donna truly believes it's important to live your authentic spiritual life and be guided to be and dwell where it *makes your soul sing.*

For further information and resources,

CONNECT WITH DONNA:

Email: sharingjoys@gmail.com

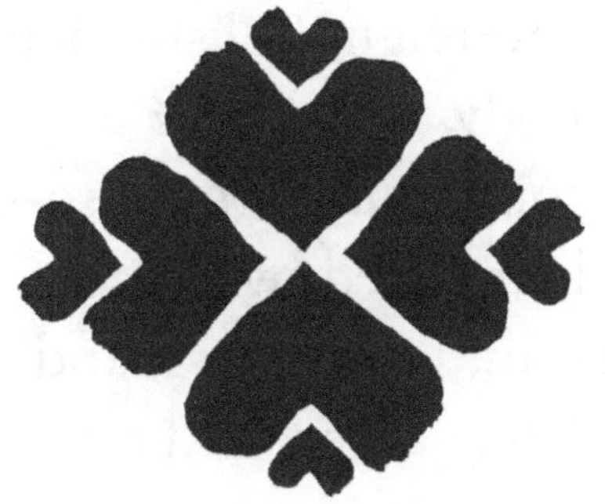

Wholeness is a state of recognizing and accepting yourself as a sovereign, holistic being composed of heart, body, mind, and soul. It means becoming conscious of those so-called flaws previously demonized by your ego-mind, and using compassion, forgiveness, and unconditional love to liberate, accept, and reintegrate them into your being.

~ David D McLeod

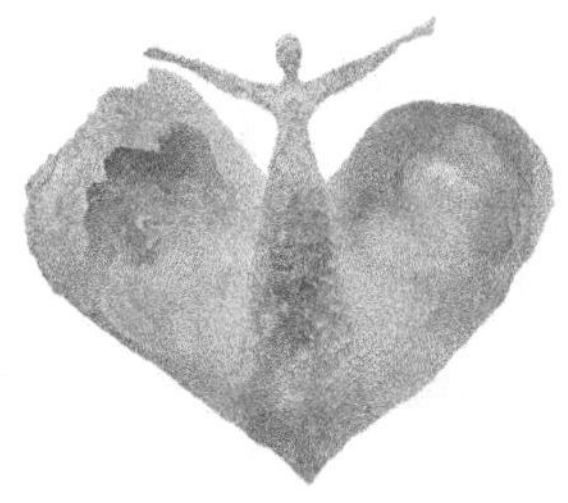

CHAPTER 12

WINDSHIELD IN THE WEEDS
A CRASH COURSE IN SELF-ACCEPTANCE

David D McLeod

DD, PHD, CERTIFIED MASTER LIFE COACH

MY STORY

BETWEEN TWO TREES

Cruise Control. 65 mph. Six feet off the ground.

Not exactly textbook driving—but that's where I found myself at 4:30 pm on August 11, 2013, in Belmont, California.

Moments earlier, I had been cruising homeward on Highway 280 in my red Hyundai Sonata, music playing, sun warming the car. The road curved left—but the car never completed the turn.

Have you ever nodded off while driving? It's happened to me a few times in my life. I don't really notice it's happening until my head jerks up, my body tightens, my eyes widen, and I thank God—or whoever is listening—that the road is still in front of me and I still have the vehicle under control. And then of course, adrenaline kicks in, and I start panting like I just sprinted the Boston Marathon.

But not this time. Somehow, everything faded rapidly to black, and I popped out in an alien world—time slowed, sounds warped.

Screee! Ch-ch-ch! Thwak!

Green and brown shapes flickered outside the windows; tree limbs thrashed the exterior. Unbeknownst to me, the car had left the road, hurtling through bushes at freeway speed. Terror seized me—until a deep, disembodied, commanding voice boomed:

"REEEELAAAAAX!"

In my crazy mind-warp, it seemed I had all the time in the world. As I pondered my circumstances, I settled on three options:

1. *Panic:* wrestle the car to a stop.

2. *Reason:* obey the reverberating voice.

3. *Uncertainty:* waffle, wait, and see.

External visibility was nonexistent, so option one was out. I've always believed that any decision is better than no decision, so option three was out, too.

I shrugged, closed my eyes, dropped my hands into my lap, and surrendered.

Okay, Captain Loudmouth, it's up to you now. Take it away.

Instantly, reality snapped back. The car whipped through branches, the side airbag detonated beside my ear, then *WHAM!*—followed by an eerie stillness.

Apparently, somewhere in my alien world, I lost the power to breathe. A frozen gasp, held for what seemed an eternity, burst out of me in a shuddering rush. The first inhale that followed flooded my body. I savored the cool and dusty air that filled my lungs—and the grateful relief that accompanied it.

Somehow, the engine was still running, so I casually flipped the ignition.

"You okay?"

"Huh?" My head jerked to the right. A vaguely familiar man in a hoodie looked down at me over the open sunroof. Concern wrinkled his face.

Is he the one who bellowed at me? I wondered. *Nah, that's ridiculous! I'm all alone here.*

I looked down at my hands and checked what I could see of myself inside the car. "Well," I said, "no blood, no broken bones. Aside from the car wreckage, everything's hunky-dory." A nervous chuckle escaped from my mouth.

When I turned back to resume the conversation, he was gone. *That was weird!* I thought, but there was something *déjà vu* about it.

The foliage-wrapped windshield sported a spiderweb of cracks but was otherwise intact. Both doors refused to open, so I squirmed my way out through the sunroof.

As soon as I stood up on the seat, I saw them twenty yards behind the car: two massive oak trees, exactly one car-width apart. Vertical white gashes scarred their trunks. I blinked, shook my head, and looked again. The gashes were a good six feet off the ground! My jaw dropped: I had sailed between them!

Holy shit! If the car had been half an inch to either side. . .

The thought trailed off, and I shuddered at the prospect. Tears erupted—fear, shock, relief, overwhelming gratitude.

Out of nowhere, a firetruck appeared on the scene. EMTs checked me over and made sure I was okay to leave. A tow truck hauled away the crumpled remnants of my vehicle. A wave of horror and sadness washed over me when I realized that a young deer had perished when the car slammed into the ground.

My friend Bob arrived. Staring at the wreckage and shaking his head, he exclaimed, "You walked away from *that?!*"

At the emergency room, the doctor was succinct. "No apparent whiplash or concussion, no internal injuries. Heart rate and blood pressure mildly elevated. You'll probably experience stress symptoms over the next few days, but we don't need to keep you. No prescriptions necessary, although you might need some Tylenol. Other than that, you're good to go. Any questions?"

In my disoriented state, I just shrugged and shook my head absently. "Thanks for checking me over." I nodded weakly to the doctor and nurse who attended to me, grabbed my backpack, and joined my friend in the waiting room.

"So what the hell happened?" Bob asked as he drove me back to my apartment.

"Still trying to figure it out," I shrugged. In that moment, no explanation seemed credible.

DECIPHERING THE MESSAGE(S)

For the next few weeks, a deep sense of wonder and awe accompanied me everywhere. There was something at play that was way bigger than I could comprehend.

Until the accident, I had seen my life journey as something designed to give me a lived and felt experience of remembering the truth of who I really am. My soul also seemed intent on guiding me to share this wisdom with the world, but my ego-mind downplayed that part of the message and supplanted my soul-desire with self-criticism and doubt.

Who are you to share such an important truth with the world? There are plenty of gurus, teachers, and leaders out there who are far more enlightened than you are!

If not for the miracle of my aliveness after the car wreck, I might've never realized that thoughts like these swam in the undercurrent of my awareness for some time, quietly suppressing the desires of my soul.

Thankfully, the Universe delivered a memo I couldn't possibly ignore. While I would gladly have skipped the car-crash component of the message, I came to realize that this form of communication was necessary for me because I had allowed my ego-mind to obstruct my understanding of my true nature. Only a proverbial "two-by-four to the back of the head" would be enough to wake me up!

By October, I decoded most of the Universe's information and flagged several important points:

1. Two sturdy oak trees were perfectly positioned in the path of my trajectory, and something literally guided my hapless vehicle right between them at exactly the right angle. This was a clear miracle, and a strong message that something or someone was protecting me. My realization that the car had actually *flown* through the air was a powerful reminder of how out of control I really was.

2. The young deer's demise signaled that a death was supposed to occur at that time. The deer served as a sacrificial substitute for me. I believe its death represented a form of divine intervention, where an innocent life was taken to spare mine.

3. I also came to see the deer as a messenger of gentleness, intuition, vulnerability, and the ability to move through life's challenges with grace. I took this as an invitation to rein in some of my more overt masculine qualities and begin embracing some of my inner feminine attributes.

4. The hooded man, who appeared out of nowhere to check on me, triggered memories that took a couple of weeks to register in my awareness. I realized I'd seen him (or felt his presence) in previous situations where I faced potential danger. As more of these memories arose, I thought things like *guardian angel* and wondered if there was a way for me to speak to this "being" directly.

5. In the short time after this incident, I noticed trees wherever I went. I recognized my deep connection to trees as individuals, but even more to nature as a whole. My sense of oneness grew stronger in my awareness, and I began to experience myself as both cause and effect—something that didn't make sense to me logically, but felt intrinsically true at my core.

6. The Universe was clearly telling me something that my human mind had difficulty accepting. But my soul was dancing with

delight—even though my body experienced this as a mixture of fear and joy. I was being instructed—in a powerful but subtle way—that my path would lead me to important work, that something greater was in store for me, that it was time for me to rise above my deeply ingrained self-limiting beliefs and bring my unique form of wisdom to the world.

The incredible bottom-line takeaway for me was that there was *something important* for me to do here, and, apparently, I hadn't yet achieved a level of self-acceptance that would open the way for me to do it. In other words, I had more inner work to do!

The Tool

Introduction

As part of the human journey, we all develop ego-minds skilled at identifying and pointing out what is wrong with us. Wellness providers and coaches often reframe this by suggesting that the ego-mind, in its own way, is trying to protect us and keep us safe. While there may be some truth to this, I believe that dwelling incessantly on flaws is incompatible with happiness and fulfillment.

Persistent focus on faults, foibles, and limitations encourages us to disown the parts of ourselves we deem inappropriate or unacceptable. We end up investing enormous amounts of energy hiding or denying these traits, eventually coming to see ourselves as broken and unworthy.

Without some form of *divine intervention,* the only way out of this convoluted self-image is self-healing—the fundamental process of restoring ourselves to wholeness.

You might ask, "What, then, is wholeness?"

Wholeness is a state of recognizing and accepting yourself as a sovereign, holistic being composed of heart, body, mind, and soul. It means becoming conscious of those so-called flaws previously demonized by your ego-mind, and using compassion, forgiveness, and unconditional love to liberate, accept, and reintegrate them into your being.

This is a profound undertaking. It demands courage—a willingness to look deeply within and uncover your truth. It may be intimidating at first, but as you likely know, even the deepest shame can be healed under the compassionate light of unconditional love.

So wrap yourself in a blanket of bravery, and join me as we explore the power of "radical self-acceptance."

THE PRACTICE

My technique is organized into three phases: (1) data-gathering, (2) analysis and reframing, and (3) mirror work. I strongly encourage you to complete all phases—avoid any temptation to take shortcuts, as this will deprive you of the full benefit of the practice.

PHASE 1. DATA GATHERING

Start by becoming intimately familiar with your ego-mind and its messages. This phase requires time and patience. I recommend dedicating at least three days to it; a full week is even better if you can manage it.

Carry a journal with you throughout your day. Proceed with your normal routine, but remain attentive to that "nasty inner voice" and its commentary about you.

As soon as you notice the internal dialogue, pause what you're doing. Open your journal and record the exact wording of the stream of thoughts. Refrain from judging or arguing with the content—simply capture it verbatim. Simultaneously, note the emotions you experience as you hear these messages.

Think of yourself as a neutral court reporter: your task is to document what you observe, hear, and feel, without internalizing or becoming attached to any of it.

PHASE 2. ANALYSIS AND REFRAMING

For this phase, set aside at least an hour in a quiet, distraction-free space. Remove all electronic devices from the space and keep only your journal and pen nearby. Choose a comfortable spot where you can sit and write. Gentle ambient music or the soft glow of candles can help create a sacred, supportive atmosphere.

1. Begin with a quiet declaration of your identity and set a clear intention. For example, you might say, "I am a divine, magnificent, unlimited, sovereign spiritual being of light and love. My intention is to open this space for holistic healing, so I may love myself unconditionally and accept myself completely." Choose words that resonate for you.

2. Take several deep, centering breaths to anchor yourself in the present moment. As you breathe, invite any sacred energies you wish to support you. Feel your innate courage blossom within, and allow a sense of excitement to grow as you embark on this healing process.

3. Sit comfortably and open your journal to the first page of ego-mind statements. Affirm out loud: "These statements emerged from my ego-mind, which seeks to protect me. I now call upon my higher self to discover the wisdom within them and reframe each into a positive affirmation to guide me forward."

4. Read the first statement out loud. Observe how it makes you feel, and grant yourself full permission to experience that emotion. Acknowledge any judgments about the statement or yourself, then consciously release them into the surrounding silence.

5. Ask yourself: "What unacknowledged truth does this statement reveal about me?" For instance, if the ego-mind statement was, "You are a lazy bum," which appears purely judgmental on the surface, search for its hidden meaning. Perhaps it indicates that you value efficiency and seek ways to simplify tasks. Isn't that a strength?

    a. Reframe it as: "I always look for ways to make life easier for myself and others."

    b. Or: "I care deeply about people and strive to reduce burdens."

    c. Or: "I engage my creativity to find inspiring, efficient solutions."

6. For every reframe, declare aloud: "**I love** this about myself!"

7. Repeat steps 4 through 6 for every message on your list. Aim to reframe each original statement into **at least two** positive, uplifting, and life-affirming truths.

Open a new journal page and compile all your reframed statements into a fresh list. Title it vibrantly: "Things I LOVE About Myself!"

By the end of this phase, you will have a substantial list of qualities you admire—far outnumbering the initial criticisms.

I call this technique *hyperlisting* because it consistently generates more positives than negatives. *Hyperlisting* can be adapted to address any personal challenge, working wonders for nurturing radical self-acceptance.

Remember, your ego-mind won't cease its chatter overnight. However, by catching its comments as they arise and reframing them immediately, you can diminish its influence and perhaps even grow to appreciate its protective intent.

PHASE 3. MIRROR, MIRROR

You've laid a strong foundation for self-acceptance. Now it's time to embody and anchor this truth. You already sense your magnificence within; this is your opportunity to acknowledge and embrace it.

Find a quiet room with a mirror—begin with a hand or wall mirror if preferred. Bring your journal.

1. Stand or sit before the mirror and gaze directly at your reflection. Relax your facial expression and allow a gentle, kind smile to form.

2. Say aloud, "I love you." Initial discomfort is natural; persist. You are worthy of love, and no one deserves your love more than you do. Repeat it with varying inflection, tone, and volume: "I love you. I love you. I love you." Continue until you begin to believe yourself.

3. Open your journal to your "Things I LOVE About Myself!" list. Select one statement that resonates and proclaim it aloud. For example, "I care about people so much that I want to make life easier all around. I **love** that about myself."

4. Repeat step three with two or three additional statements, concluding each with ". . .and I love that about myself."

5. Complete the practice by looking yourself in the eyes, wrapping your arms around yourself in a loving embrace, and affirming, "I accept all of you. I love you."

6. Return tomorrow and do the exercise again, this time using different statements from your affirmation list.

With regular practice, this will feel increasingly natural. To intensify the experience, try performing this ritual naked before a full-length mirror—its power is transformative.

FINAL WORDS

Here is a daily mantra I use to remain grounded in my truth, expressed with gratitude for every aspect of my being:

- I gratefully forgive the imperfect being I have been in the past.

- I gratefully accept the magnificent being I am right now.

- I gratefully welcome the evolved being I am becoming in each new moment.

Self-acceptance is the root of self-love; you cannot truly love yourself without fully accepting yourself. And self-healing is necessary if you wish to develop and enhance self-acceptance. Take the time to honor who you are and bring yourself back to wholeness. Grant yourself permission to recognize and embrace the truly amazing being you are—and experience true happiness and fulfillment in the bargain!

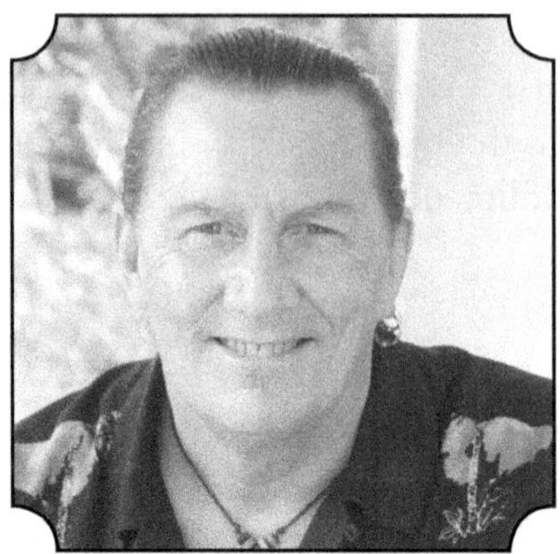

David McLeod is an award-winning #1 international bestselling author and master life coach who guides men and women beyond limiting beliefs into the fullness of their God-given potential. His work is a unique synthesis of disciplined logic and creative insight, forged in the crucible of a remarkable life.

A former fighter pilot and software engineer, David understands the world of structure, strategy, and intellect. As a poet, musician, and artist, he is equally fluent in the language of intuition, heart, and creative expression. This rare duality allows him to speak to the whole person—addressing both the mind that seeks answers and the soul that seeks meaning.

David is a proud father, a perpetual student, and a humble teacher. He brings a wealth of lived experience—not just theory—to his work as a transformational speaker, coach, and storyteller. His mission is clear: to provide others with the practical skills and profound clarity needed to build a life of authentic purpose, unshakeable peace, and passionate vitality.

David holds a PhD in Metaphysical Sciences and a Doctorate in Holistic Personal Coaching, further solidifying the extensive expertise he brings to his practice. He empowers people worldwide to become true masters of their lives, turning daily challenges into opportunities for profound growth and lasting victory.

CONNECT WITH DAVID:

Website: https://yourlifemasterycoach.com

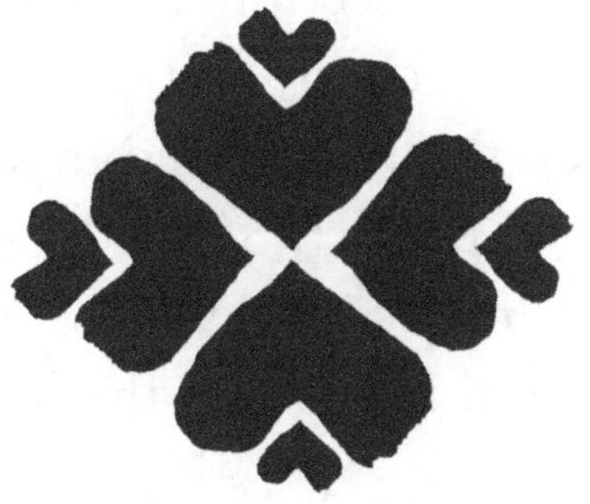

My body whispered for years—headaches, tightness in my chest, and fainting—but I pushed through, determined to keep our life looking picture perfect. Stress doesn't just sit in your mind; it moves in, decorates your nervous system, and rearranges the furniture.

~ Jane Ann Guyette

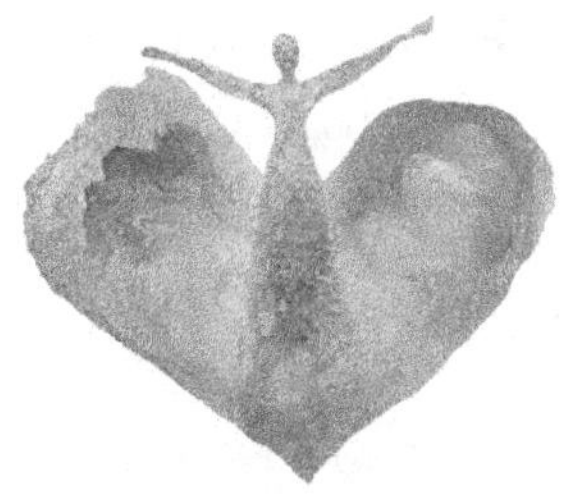

CHAPTER 13

It's All in Your Head
Breathing Beyond the Stories That Bind You

Jane Ann Guyette

CHT., Author, Yoga Teacher, BS

My Story

Why won't you look me in the eyes? Something's wrong.

It started with just one look. It was all I needed. I knew in that still place inside me that never lies.

He traveled often, but this time, when he came home, something was different. No kiss. Just a side hug, the kind you give your aunt at Thanksgiving, not your wife after two weeks apart.

His focus was on the kids. He brushed past me, and the air froze between us. I knew it was more than travel fatigue. Weeks of subtle shifts, sighs, silences, and the way my laugh seemed to irritate him prepared me for what I soon found.

That night, I celebrated his return home, grateful to have him back, but the next day, something inside me needed answers. I followed the ache in my chest as if it were a compass, leading me straight to the truth. He guarded his phone, so I turned to his computer. There, I discovered an unfamiliar email account under a different name, along with saved passwords linked to it. When I opened the account, I noticed a message from "Ashley Madison." Curious, I searched the name, thinking she was a real person, maybe a coworker. *Wrong!* It turned out to be a dating website known for connecting married individuals seeking affairs, using the slogan: "Life is short. Have an affair."

I confronted him. "What the hell is this?"

"My friends told me about it and I was curious," he replied. He looked me in the eyes and said, "I swear nothing is going on. You're overreacting. This is all in your head!"

A couple of years later, that same uneasy feeling crept back, and the heaviness in my stomach told me something wasn't right. I couldn't ignore it. So, once again, I searched. I found an email thread with a woman he met at a conference. The messages were filled with familiarity, laughter, and words that left no doubt they were close. One line burned into my mind. "I can't wait to get back to Carson City to be with you again." My heart folded in on me, the beating of it deafening. I felt the air leave the room, and with it the last bit of safety I knew. I called him, voice trembling, "I saw the emails."

He worked over an hour away, yet somehow he was home in less than half an hour, pleading, "I swear it's nothing, please forgive me." But as he stood there, desperate and full of excuses, my heart didn't just break; it fractured the world we built around it.

We had young children, and I still believed in us. Counseling gave me hope. "Marriages survive this," our therapist said, and for a while ours did, but it was different. Anything that gave me a sense of purpose or control, he slowly began to take over.

Leading the Women's Club was a source of joy, a place where I felt seen, heard, and genuinely useful. But each time I mentioned it, he sighed, "You do too much for everyone else, Jane, and for what? It's not even paid." Out of guilt and love, I stepped down. Something inside me shifted, and the space between us widened. One day, I glanced at my calendar, once filled with color-coded plans, and found it empty.

Little by little, the life we built together began to unravel. I didn't see it then, but control can often disguise itself as concern. His work always came first, and I became invisible, my world shrinking around me until I was just a shadow of who I once was.

I saw a picture of her, the other woman on social media. She was much thinner. Unaware, I began molding myself in her image and, in doing so, disappeared. I withered away, dropping to 95 pounds at 5'6." My jeans hung loose on my hips. Meals and conversations faded into bites and nods. I felt small and unseen. One morning, brushing my hair, I noticed how dull my eyes looked, as if someone dimmed the brightness inside me.

Why am I not enough?

My body was the messenger, headaches, tightness in my chest, even fainting—but I was determined to keep our life looking picture perfect. Stress doesn't just sit in your mind; it moves in, decorates your nervous system, and rearranges the furniture.

One day, my body said what I couldn't—"No more!" I had my first grand mal seizure, which wouldn't stop with meds, and ended up in the hospital for a week.

I woke as if I had been ripped from another dimension, my body here, but my soul still catching up. The lights were so bright my eyes wouldn't stop watering, my body trembled, my hands refused to unclench, and every muscle was heavy with exhaustion. My mind was blank in places where memories used to be. The days blurred together; I couldn't remember conversations, faces, or even moments that should've anchored me. It was terrifying, not knowing what I had lost, yet beneath the fear, something stirred. My body spoke the only way it knew how; it seized.

That seizure wasn't just a collapse, but a calling, my body's way of shaking me awake, grasping what my heart refused to acknowledge, saying, "If you won't seize the day, I will."

In the quiet that followed, I realized it wasn't just about what happened to me; it was about what needed to change within me.

After my first seizure, there was a shift in my husband's eyes, an unspoken blame that made me feel like a burden. I didn't fight or flee,

I fawned. We often hear about fight or flight, yet rarely about the third response: fawn, the instinct to become small and appease.

The medication's side effects sank me into a darkness I didn't know existed.

Will this fog ever lift?

My spirit shattered, I clawed at the emptiness, searching for a trace of feeling.

Maybe I'll save enough of these until I have enough to leave this Earth.

Ironically, that plan ended up saving my life.

As I tapered off the medication, fragments of myself began to return, like sunlight through heavy clouds. That glimmer of clarity sent me on a new search for a medication that wouldn't steal my mind while trying to save my body. I tried at least five different prescriptions. At one point, I joked that I was personally keeping the pharmaceutical industry afloat. Each new bottle came with side effects: fatigue, fog, forgetfulness. Eventually, I found one I could tolerate, though it came with a hefty price tag. Days after a seizure, I learned my insurance had denied coverage due to the cost. What followed was a marathon of phone calls, paperwork, and pleading with strangers to understand that this wasn't about convenience, it was about survival. Every refill became a small battle, and each two-week wait for approval was filled with anxiety, hope, and the kind of patience only chronic illness can teach.

My anxiety became its own illness. Once, after a terrible seizure that landed me in the emergency room again, I couldn't risk waiting. When my insurance denied the only drug that helped, I paid out of pocket, $8000 just to stay alive—$8000!

Trying to get reimbursed was a nightmare; each call began with hold music. I retold my story, over and over. "I understand," they'd say, then passed me on to another person who couldn't help. By the fifth insurance rep, I wasn't Jane anymore; I was policy number 429-B. It wasn't just exhausting, it was dehumanizing. I never did get reimbursed, no reason given, just denied.

The constant battles for my health mirrored the ones unfolding in my home—both draining, both unsustainable.

Our marriage didn't survive, but perhaps that was a hidden grace. Had I stayed, I might have lost not only myself, but my life.

How do I get out of this hole?

The truth was, I couldn't think my way out. I was too medicated to feel, and too exhausted to fight. So my body erupted in the only language it knew, seizures. Each new drug promised relief but stole another piece of me. Some made me so sick I could hardly move; others pulled me into such darkness I no longer wanted to be here.

With my doctor's help, I slowly weaned off eight pills a day until the fog began to lift. That's when I realized: it didn't matter whether I took medication or not, the seizures still came.

At least now I wasn't poisoning myself to survive, and I could feel again, even if it was pain. The feelings and tears came without warning. I wailed. The sound that left me didn't even feel human. I touched my chest and didn't want the feeling to stop. The ache was proof that I was still here, still capable of feeling anything at all. My body wasn't the enemy; it was the messenger. Every seizure, every symptom, was its way of pleading with me to wake up, reclaim my life, and live differently.

NOTE TO MY READERS:

According to my neurologist, once you have epilepsy, you will always have it. One in twenty-six people will experience a seizure at some point in their lives, and there is no known cure. My neurologist told me that stress does not cause seizures. Maybe not in textbooks, but my body never read those chapters. The day I was served divorce papers, mine spoke, in the only language it knew, a full-blown seizure, and again on the day I filed them. "All in your head," he said without looking up from his computer. The next time, I asked my family to record one. After seeing the video, my doctor went quiet. He confirmed it was a grand mal seizure, not imagined. That moment taught me that even experts can be wrong. While epilepsy may never fully disappear, I've learned that through self-awareness, stress management, and intentional healing, its power over your life can greatly diminish.

"At least it's just epilepsy."

That's what someone said to me after I was hospitalized for a severe episode, six hours of seizures, repeated head trauma, and a mild heart attack.

"Just epilepsy." *As if it were a mild inconvenience, like losing Wi-Fi or running out of coffee.*

When I came to, I had no memory of the previous six months. My body ached as if I had been dragged behind a car down a dirt road. In connection with that, with every seizure, I lost my license for six months, which makes it nearly impossible to work, run errands, or have a social life.

In some ways, it was even harder on my loved ones. I didn't remember who they were, and sometimes, I didn't even remember who I was. I spent days scrolling through my phone, emails, and photos, trying to piece together the missing months of my life. *What have I been doing? What responsibilities have I forgotten?* Then there's the fear, the quiet, ever-present dread that it will happen again. You never know when, or if, but it lingers like a shadow that never leaves the room. I stopped saying yes to things—to people, to plans, to life—because there are no warning signs for me, and for many with epilepsy—no flashing lights. No sirens. Just silence, and then the fall.

That's the hidden side of epilepsy, the one no one sees, and few understand.

After countless MRIs and EEGs, the doctors traced my seizures back to a head injury I sustained in second grade. We played Crack the Whip on the playground when I was thrown into the side of the school, knocked unconscious for hours, and rushed to the emergency room. I don't remember the impact, only my mother's face, her eyes wide and filled with fear. I knew something was seriously wrong.

Years later, during a painful divorce, that old head injury resurfaced physically, emotionally, and energetically. It was in that space of unraveling and in the quiet after a seizure that I discovered the only thing I could control, my breath. One inhale. One exhale. That's where I began. Over time, I learned to weave the power of hypnosis and breathwork together, two forces that helped me heal from the inside out.

Awareness may open the door, but healing requires action.

So I created a tool that helped me heal from seizures, heartache, betrayal, and the many layers of pain that come with trauma and divorce.

THE TOOL

RETURNING TO YOURSELF: A GUIDED PRACTICE

Before you begin, put on soft music and take a quiet moment to check in with yourself.

Open your journal and, without judgment, write a few words or short phrases about your current state.

ASK YOURSELF:

- How does my body feel right now? Example: tense shoulders, tight chest, heavy stomach.

- What emotions are most present? Example: anxious, numb, peaceful, sad.

- What thoughts or worries are looping in my mind?

- On a scale of 1–10, how connected do I feel to myself? 1 = disconnected, 10 = fully aligned.

SETTLING IN

Find a peaceful space where you won't be disturbed. Sit or lie down comfortably with your hands and feet uncrossed.

Take three deep letting-go breaths, in through the nose, out through the mouth.

Gently focus your gaze on a single point on the ceiling. Stare at that spot until you feel your eyes tire. With each slow blink, feel them grow heavier until they naturally close.

Feel your eyelids resting heavily, comfortably. Allow that relaxation to spread through your face, your shoulders, your chest, all the way down through your legs and feet. Let it radiate through you completely, calm, warm, and peaceful.

Descending into Calm

Now, imagine a beautiful staircase before you.

With each step downward, feel yourself moving deeper into ease and comfort.

At the bottom is a door to a special place, a sanctuary of peace and safety. Open it and step inside.

Here, every breath settles your body.

Your shoulders loosen. Your jaw releases.

You drift inward, deeper into stillness, deeper into yourself.

The Breath

Bring your awareness to your breath.

Inhale for a count of **four,** hold for **two,** exhale for **six.**

Repeat for five rounds, then return to a natural rhythm.

With each exhale, feel tension melting away.

Let your breath move like a wave, washing through you, cleansing, softening, and releasing all that no longer serves you.

The Heart and the Knower

Place one hand over your heart and one over your solar plexus, your center of truth and power.

Feel the gentle rhythm beneath your palms and silently repeat in your mind:

"With every breath, I return to myself."

"With every exhale, I release what is not mine."

Now, imagine a soft golden light glowing in your heart. Let it expand, filling your body, your mind, and your energy field. This light is your self-love awakening.

It knows how to heal and guide you home.

Breathe that golden light into any place holding pain or tightness, physical or emotional.

See the light swirling, softening, transforming.

"With every breath, I forgive myself and others."

"With every breath, I awaken to love."

Repeat as often as feels right.

RETURNING

Stay here as long as you need.

When you're ready, take one final deep letting-go breath, releasing the past and reclaiming your power.

Gently open your eyes.

Feel the calm, wholeness, and connection returning to you.

You've come home to your breath, your body, and yourself.

REFLECTION

Afterward, take a few minutes to journal:

- How do I feel in my body now?

- How do I feel emotionally?

- Did I experience release, relief, or expansion?

- What shifted, and was it subtle or significant?

- What am I most grateful for in this moment?

These prompts help anchor your insights into daily life, revealing that people don't disappoint you; your expectations do.

Betrayal is rarely one-sided. It grows in the corners of a marriage, in the moments we stop showing up for each other, where love gets lost behind responsibility and routine.

Neither of us was perfect. We carried our own faults, past traumas, addictions, and insecurities, each one shaping the dysfunction between us. No one was entirely to blame. Life's a classroom, and that relationship was one hell of a lesson. It taught me I'd been living for everyone but me. Now, I choose alignment over approval.

In losing my marriage and my health, I lost the illusion of control, but I gained a deeper connection to life itself.

Hypnotic breathwork became my compass, guiding me from survival into presence. It showed me that healing isn't about fixing what's broken, but remembering what's whole.

Through this practice, with each breath, I felt pieces return, a softness in my voice, a steadiness in my demeanor, a spark behind my eyes. I was no longer surviving. I was remembering. Each conscious breath invites you to soften pain, release what no longer serves you, and reconnect with your wisdom within. This practice isn't about escaping your story; it's about transforming it from the inside out.

As you breathe with awareness, you awaken the part of you that already knows how to heal, how to trust, and how to begin again.

I'm doing it, you can too!

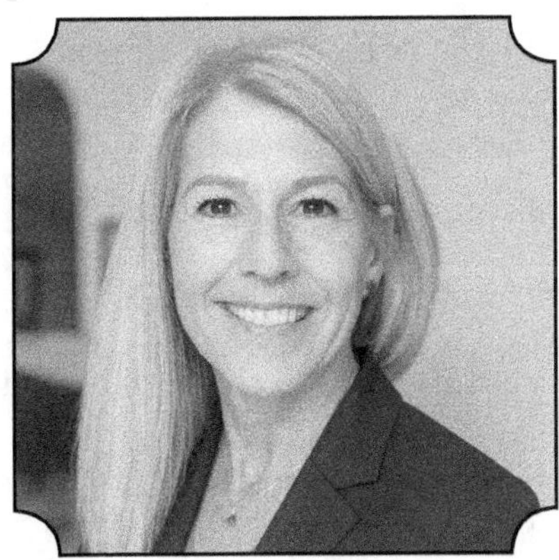

Jane Ann Guyette, C.Ht.

Jane Ann Guyette helps clients restore balance in body, mind, and soul through hypnosis and energy work, guiding them to access subconscious wisdom, release old patterns, and create lasting transformation.

She is a certified clinical hypnotherapist, best-selling author, dietitian, public speaker, yoga instructor, Reiki Master, and the founder of Alive2Thrive Hypnosis.

A graduate of the Clinical Hypnosis Institute of Michigan, Jane specializes in whole-heart healing, self-hypnosis, anxiety, and weight management. Whether you're seeking relief, renewal, or rebirth, Jane meets you where you are and helps you find the peace that's been waiting within you all along.

Before founding Alive2Thrive Hypnosis, Jane spent years in clinical settings. Her degree in dietetics from the University of Wisconsin Stevens Point gave her the scientific foundation for understanding the body, but her passion for energy, movement, and the subconscious revealed the missing link: healing doesn't begin in the body; it starts in the mind.

Today, Jane's clients and audiences describe her as a transformational presence, a voice of clarity who helps people access their innate healing abilities. Whether she's teaching self-hypnosis, speaking to a crowd, or working one-on-one, her mission is to support your journey toward deep, lasting healing. Change your mind, Change your life.

Awaken the part of you that's ready to thrive, Fully Alive!

Connect with Jane Ann:

Email: Alive2thrivehypnosis@gmail.com

Website: https://www.alive2thrivehypnosis.com/

Facebook: https://www.facebook.com/intuitivejane/

YouTube: http://www.youtube.com/@alive2thriveinabundance456

My Tool: Listen to a guided hypnosis on YouTube:
https://www.youtube.com/watch?v=FmN7iHLj0r8

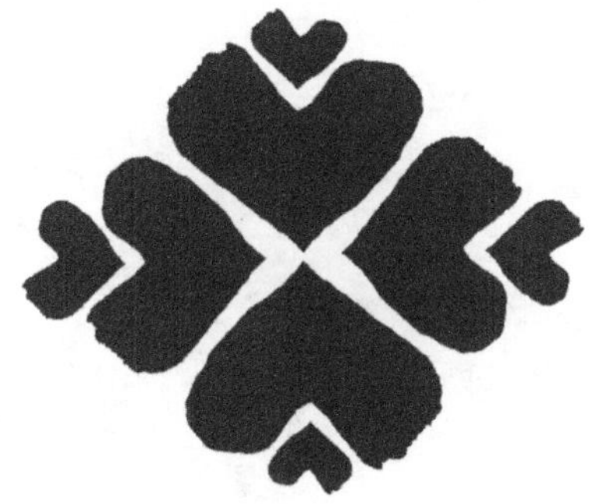

NERVOUS SYSTEM HEALING

Everything I knew said this couldn't happen. But it just had. If this is possible, what else am I wrong about?

~ Johanna Farrimond

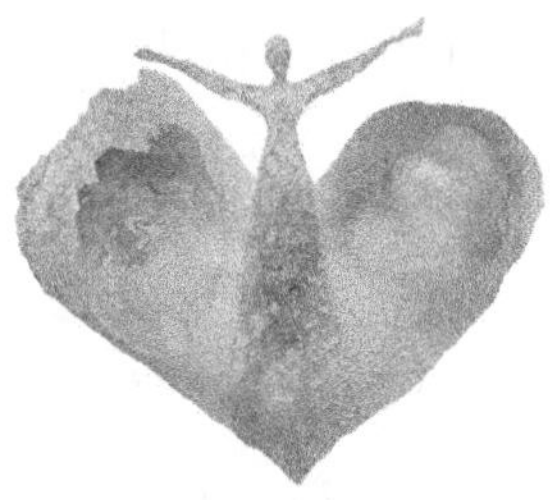

Chapter 14

Your Burnout Isn't Psychological; It's Energetic

Clearing the Bioelectric Blockage Therapy Can't Touch

Johanna Farrimond

M.S.

You work eighteen-hour days to feel nothing. Success feels hollow. Decisions paralyze you. Your razor-sharp mind went dark. Everything you've tried—therapy, meditation, holidays—nothing works. Because burnout isn't psychological, it's an electrical failure. And no amount of mindset work can restart a dead circuit.

My Story

I sat at the intersection staring at the sign. *Psychic Readings. Walk-ins Welcome.* It was the same corner I'd driven past for a year, the same sign I pretended not to see.

The light turned green. I didn't move. The car behind me honked. I turned anyway.

Rock bottom looks different for everyone. Mine was a psychic's storefront on a Tuesday afternoon.

I went in. Inside, incense hung thick enough to taste. Everything exactly as you'd expect from a strip-mall mystic. The woman across from me shuffled cards with practiced precision while I tried to formulate my question in a way that didn't sound completely pathetic.

"I need to make a career decision," I managed.

She studied my face. Not the cards. Me. Her eyes narrowed. 'Any choice is fine. There's no right or wrong answer."

I handed her two twenties and walked out. Slouched in my car and finally admitted what I denied for months:

I can't feel my decisions anymore.

Every answer feels the same. Wrong.

The Descent

It began in the middle of the night. Not with quiet breaths, but with a thudding alarm deep in my chest, pulse pounding like a heavy fist. My mind ran attack scenarios:

What if we fail our security assessment? Have we done enough to protect against an insider threat?

I drafted defenses for battles that didn't exist.

Weeks later, I stood frozen in the yogurt aisle at Wegman's. Fifteen minutes. Paralyzed by choice. Every tiny decision felt like a full system breach.

Then the crunch from above—my bike, crushed against the garage ceiling, still strapped to the car roof. I just stood there, looking at the wreckage of my attention.

Your nervous system doesn't send calendar invites. It just stops. Mine started with my period vanishing for six months: no medical answers, just pills to restart the silence. Then my hair, not strands but clumps, circling the shower drain like evidence of a crime.

After a staff meeting, my boss pulled me aside. "You've got monkey mind," he said, not unkindly. Perfect diagnosis. Forty-seven browser tabs, all frozen, all screaming "Threat!"

Then came Hashimoto's. My immune system was attacking my thyroid like a foreign invader. My body declared war on itself.

When the promotion came—Cyber Advisor to the Deputy Assistant Secretary of Defense—I stared at that offer letter for three weeks. Printed it. Highlighted it. Made pro/con lists. Four pages. Asked everyone. Inside, a record skipped:

You don't deserve this.

The harder I tried to think clearly, the murkier everything became. That's how I ended up at the psychic's table, hoping mysticism could fix what logic couldn't.

THE GEOGRAPHIC CURE (THAT WASN'T)

That week, I quit. It felt like control. Everyone said it was brave. I'd sell everything. Move to Maui.

If I remove the pressure and live in paradise, my system will reset.

Six months later, at a conference, I met Neil—British accent, kind eyes. We talked until the early morning, and for the first time in months, the world softened. My company approved a UK transfer instead of Maui. Three weeks after moving, we flew to Vegas, took a helicopter over the Grand Canyon, and got married.

Fresh start, right? But the moment the champagne fizzed, the doubts arrived.

What if this is just escapism? What if I've made a terrible mistake?

The catastrophic thinking packed itself in my luggage, cleared customs, and set up shop in our Eton flat with a view of Windsor Castle.

My left shoulder locked first. I woke up and could barely lift my arm. "Adhesive capsulitis," the doctor said. My body built its own prison. Months of physical therapy and acupuncture barely made a dent.

Then carpal tunnel struck. My hand throbbed. My grip was useless. My neck followed—a sharp, stabbing pain and then, the MRI: a slipped disc pressing against my spine.

Sitting on that examination table, facing a steroid injection in my neck—one wrong move meant paralysis—I broke. Forty-two years old, thousands of miles from home, crying while my husband stood there, helpless.

That evening, my mother's voice crossed the miles. "I had a dream," she said, "that you were stuck, trapped in the UK, wondering if moving there was the biggest mistake you ever made."

Her words landed hard—a heavy mirror to my own dark thoughts.

How could she know?

"Everything's fine, Mom." But my body was screaming the truth she already dreamed.

The Portugal Prescription

"Let's move to Portugal," my husband suggested one grey November morning. "Simplify everything."

By April, we were settled in a traditional tiled house tucked into a peaceful valley. Roosters woke us at dawn. Oranges hung heavy in the yard.

This will fix everything.

Three weeks in paradise—that's how long the honeymoon lasted before my nervous system caught on, realizing there were no actual threats to manage, and started to invent its own.

What if our investments crash? What if my husband gets sick?

What if we made a terrible mistake?

3 a.m. every night—wide awake, heart pounding, mind racing through catastrophes that didn't exist, while the peaceful rush of a nearby river flowed outside our window.

Two years passed like this. I tried everything—therapy, meditation, breathwork, cold plunges. Nothing touched it. Eventually, I stopped trying—early retirement. The freedom I believed would heal me.

My body kept sending signals—night sweats, sudden hot flashes. Early menopause, I told myself. But underneath, a voice whispered:

This is who you are now.

The lightness I carried my whole life? Gone. It belonged to someone else.

THE EXPERIMENT THAT CHANGED EVERYTHING

"Remote hip alignment," my friend texted. "This has to be fake, right?"

Probably. Almost definitely. But I'd been burned by my own assumptions before. Curiosity nagged me. So instead of dismissing it, I decided to find out. Five willing expats, one bemused physical therapist, proper measurements—*let's see what actually happens.*

We met in the therapist's office. My laptop ran Zoom. My husband filmed. The healer joined from Mexico—no physical contact, no manipulation.

"Stand in front of the camera," he said. "I need to see your face. Close your eyes."

I felt nothing. No sensation. No shift. Two seconds of silence.

"It's done."

The therapist measured me first. "They're even," he said with surprise in his voice. I made him measure again. "Even." Then he measured the others. All five expats—perfectly aligned. Not subtle shifts, undeniable changes.

I stood frozen while tears leaked out—my body processing what my mind refused to accept. Everything I knew said this couldn't happen. But it just had.

If this is possible, what else am I wrong about?

Three days later, I contacted him. "Teach me."

He walked me through the hip alignment over Zoom. Clean. Systematic. Point A to Point B. I tried it on a visiting family member. Hips aligned in seconds. Then a woman in Laos—same result. The precision satisfied something in me. This protocol worked every time.

I took his courses. They were different—no specific protocols. "Energy follows attention and intention," they said. "Chase the pain." Every session became improvisation—tracking sensation, following intuition, letting energy guide me to places I couldn't see or explain.

Sometimes it worked beautifully. A friend's sciatica dissolved. My own pain often resolved quickly. But I couldn't explain what made some sessions work while others didn't. No variables to adjust. No steps to troubleshoot.

My physics training kept interrupting: *What's the mechanism? Can you repeat it?*

"Everyone's energy is unique," they explained. "Trust the process."

Trust. Intuition. Process. The words felt hollow against my need for structure.

That hip alignment technique stuck with me. Precise. Consistent. Teachable. Five tries, five hits. No exceptions.

If healing could work like that—systematic, reliable, measurable—why did everything else require mystery?

The question wouldn't let go: *If one technique can be this precise, why can't they all?*

The First Crack in the Pattern

Fast forward to June 2024. During a virtual energy-healing exchange, someone mentioned Tong Ren, a protocol developed by Tom Tam, an acupuncturist and Chi Gong master in Boston. What caught my attention: *success rates.* Actual percentages for conditions. The first time I heard healing work described as a clinical trial.

Tong Ren works by clearing bioelectrical blockages in the nervous system. My engineer mind lit up. In computer networks, disruptions in the physical layer—damaged cables, obstructed connections—cripple data flow and degrade performance. *If your body works on bioelectrical pathways, blockages might operate the same way—hardware faults, not software bugs.*

Tom Tam developed this system because traditional acupuncture and Western medicine frustrated him. Western medicine managed symptoms but rarely cured root causes. He drew on the ancient Huatuojiaji method—spinal points discovered around 200 A.D. by the physician Hua Tuo—and combined it with Western anatomy and systematic protocols, resulting in precise, repeatable interventions targeting specific blockages.

I found a free online session focused on cancer support. The Zoom chat was alive—people sharing test results, celebrating healing victories, reporting their doctors' surprise. Between updates, Tom Tam called out specific points while practitioners tapped anatomical dolls in sync.

Then I felt it—the wave of collective tapping washing through me was intense, unmistakable, like receiving a personal session through the screen.

A few days later, I joined another session, this one titled "Emotions." I lay down on the sofa, phone beside my ear. The rhythmic tap-tap-tap began, hammer on doll, point by point. A Boston accent called out coordinates, systematic and precise: "GV-twenty, now movin' to BL-six, focusin' on the fronta lobe heah. . ."

Fifteen minutes in, I drifted off to the rhythmic tapping.

THE 3 A.M. MIRACLE NOBODY BELIEVES

I woke at my usual time, 3 a.m. Right on cue, the worry arrived: What if something happens to Neil? My husband was healthy, fifty-four, with no risk factors. Yet my nervous system appointed itself his personal threat assessor, running worst-case scenarios every night at precisely 3 a.m.

I braced for the familiar cascade: adrenaline rush, disaster reels, heart pounding. But instead, my mind surprised me. It offered calm, practical solutions and settled on: If something happens, I'll handle it.

That was it—no panic, no spiral. Worry knocked, saw no one home, and left.

I got up and walked to the bathroom. Moonlight spilled through the window. Standing there, I felt something I hadn't in over a decade: calm. Not the exhausted calm after a panic attack. Not the numb calm Xanax brought. Real calm. Like my nervous system finally received the software update it begged for.

Three days later, I got my first test. I walked into our bathroom and stopped. There, in the bathtub, sat a Portuguese wolf spider—legs stretched wide, marking its territory. We looked at each other.

The old me would've panicked. But something shifted. I didn't feel fear; I felt compassion. For the first time, I saw the spider not as scary, but as scared. Gently, I scooped it into a glass and carried it outside—no rush, no adrenaline, just quiet understanding.

Two weeks later, the real test arrived. Morning coffee in hand, I opened our front gate and nearly stepped on a snake. My usual response to snakes was so dramatic. My husband had a protocol: Hear wife scream, get her inside, remove snake, provide detailed proof of removal, wait 24 hours before discussing the incident.

I stood there quietly, waiting for my nervous system's scream. But it never came. *Huh, snake. Interesting.* I stepped around it without hesitation and checked the mailbox.

It wasn't courage. I didn't grow brave overnight. The fear wasn't there to overcome. The part of my nervous system that screamed "DANGER" for over a decade finally went quiet.

WHEN THE PATTERN FINALLY BREAKS

Over the next month, I watched a decade of dysfunction quietly dismantle itself. Decisions became simple again—not always easy, but simple. The paralysis lifted. I could look at options, weigh them, and choose—no tarot cards required.

Most nights, I slept straight through for eight hours, no interruption. Occasionally, I woke around 3 a.m., but instead of panic, those moments were peaceful. I noticed I was awake, turned over, and drifted right back to sleep—no adrenaline surge, no spiraling catastrophes.

My neck and shoulders loosened slowly, incrementally, with a few more degrees of movement each week. My physical therapist was baffled. "Whatever you're doing, keep doing it." The carpal tunnel vanished, my grip strength came back, and my hot flashes stopped.

I kept waiting for the old patterns to return. They didn't.

But the most profound shift was one I didn't target: my relationship with alcohol. For years, I used wine as a manual downshift, two glasses to stop the mental spinning. Not quite alcoholism, but definitely self-medication.

One evening, months later, I uncorked a bottle of Portuguese red and realized I didn't want it, not through white-knuckle willpower, but genuine lack of desire. The craving dissolved. My nervous system found its way back to balance.

The Science I Couldn't Ignore

The engineer in me needed to understand what happened. I ordered Tom Tam's books and dove into bioelectrical theory. I studied the autonomic nervous system and found research documenting measurable results with Tong Ren: 64% anxiety reduction, 61% improvement in depression through nervous system recalibration.

My nervous system was stuck in threat detection mode for so long that it forgot any other setting existed. The blockages kept it locked in that pattern, no matter what was happening around me. That's why moving to Portugal didn't help, why retirement didn't help. Why didn't therapy help? They were all addressing the software while the hardware remained corrupted.

Every nerve in your body carries an electrical current. When blockages form—resistance in the circuit—current can't flow properly. Organs don't get the signals they need, and systems fail.

Tong Ren targets these blockage points, clears them, and restores flow.

It's debugging, essentially. But for humans instead of servers.

I spent twenty years in IT security, identifying vulnerabilities before they caused system failures. Now I've discovered the same principles applied to human nervous systems—clear the blockages, restore the function.

Two months after that first session, I enrolled in a Tong Ren certification course. I practiced. Then I began offering sessions, first to friends, then strangers, then people worldwide via Zoom. The pattern held—executives who couldn't make decisions regained clarity. Chronic pain vanished. Decades-old anxiety dissolved. Not everyone. Not everything. But enough to know this was real.

THE TOOL

TONG REN THERAPY

Here's what makes Tong Ren different from everything else I'd tried.

Your nervous system runs on electricity. Every cell maintains an electrical charge. Your neurons fire electrical signals. Your heart beats on electrical impulses. When chronic stress exhausts you, it creates blockages that scramble these pathways, like corrosion in wiring. The current can't flow properly. Signals can't reach their destinations. Systems start failing.

That's why therapy, meditation, and breathwork often can't fully resolve burnout. They address the psychological layer—the software. But they can't clear the hardware dysfunction.

Tom Tam mapped specific points along your spine and skull that directly influence your autonomic nervous system and major organs, linking these to treatable conditions. The Huatuojiaji points along your spine connect to your heart, lungs, kidneys, and other vital systems. The cranial points on your head influence brain function, hormonal balance, and emotional regulation. When these points are blocked by chronic stress or trauma, bioelectrical flow deteriorates—organs malfunction, and the nervous system stalls.

During a Tong Ren session, a practitioner taps points on a small anatomical doll with a magnetic hammer, with the doll representing the client and the tapping directing healing energy to the corresponding areas in your body.

Tong Ren systematically clears these specific blockages, restoring flow.

The mechanism remains unclear, but what's certain is that collective intention shows documented effects. Consciousness appears to operate non-locally. Most importantly, it works. The doll facilitates focused intention on precise blockage points in your body. Like debugging code remotely—you don't need physical access to the server to fix it.

What convinced me wasn't the theory. It was waking up at 3 a.m. without panic for the first time in a decade.

GETTING STARTED WITHOUT THE OVERWHELM

You don't need expertise to benefit from Tong Ren. Start wherever feels right:

Try It Yourself. Without access to the doll and hammer, you can still practice this healing method effectively. Use your fingertips to tap acupoints on a diagram. The exact locations and diagrams are available at https://tools.johanna.life to guide your practice. Start with a protocol for anxiety relief to calm an overactive nervous system. Tap at any pace that feels right, spending at least ten seconds on each point. This tapping sequence takes less than 10 minutes.

Begin with LI18 near the sides of your Adam's apple, then SI16 on the right side of your neck. Move to the crown points—GV23 and GV22 at the top of your head—to calm the nervous system. Tap GB13 on the right side, targeting the frontal lobe, then Yiming behind your ear for emotional balance. Continue to Tian Dong, where your neck meets your shoulder, increasing blood flow to the vertebral artery. Target C2 on the right side, activating the vagus nerve, then T5 on the left side of your upper spine to calm the heart. Finish with H7 at your wrist—to promote peace.

Practice on yourself or loved ones—no pressure, just exploration. Ready for your own kit? The doll, magnetic hammer, and books are at https://tongrenshop.com.

Experience It Live. Watch free group sessions online. Feel the energy in real time as you learn the protocols for specific conditions. Group sessions amplify collective intention, making effects more powerful. You can find a daily schedule here:

https://tongrenstation.com/tong-ren-healing-therapy-live-broadcast-schedule

Get Personalized Support. Schedule a one-on-one session for your specific blockages. Sixty minutes focused entirely on you. Schedule at https://johanna.life/services

The most common response after session one? "I slept better than I have in years."

Why? Tong Ren clears the bioelectrical blockages anchoring your sympathetic nervous system in overdrive. Your body suddenly remembers how to rest.

You don't need to understand electricity to flip a switch. The body knows what to do once energy flows.

Your curiosity is enough.

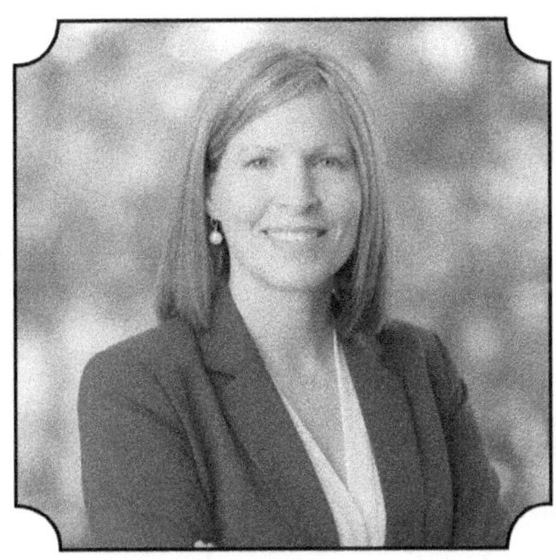

Johanna Farrimond spent twenty years in consulting and security, including more than a decade supporting the Department of Defense, where she rose to Head of Security and Risk Management for a classified government network, safeguarding continuity of operations at the highest levels of government. She knew how to protect against every conceivable threat, except the one that came from inside her own nervous system. When chronic burnout manifested as Hashimoto's disease, frozen shoulder, and catastrophic thinking that followed her through three country moves and early retirement, conventional medicine offered no solutions. Therapy helped her understand the problem, and medication managed symptoms, but neither addressed the bioelectrical dysfunction at the root.

Her analytical training made her the perfect skeptic. She recorded an experiment to debunk energy healing, complete with a physical therapist and other skeptics. When five people's hips aligned measurably over Zoom, documented on video, her certainty about what was possible shattered. That crack in her worldview led her to Tong Ren therapy, where she discovered that nervous system dysfunction wasn't psychological but bioelectrical. One session targeting emotional blockages dissolved the catastrophic thinking pattern that had haunted her for over a decade.

The engineer in her recognized something familiar in Tom Tam's Tong Ren framework: systematic diagnosis, repeatable protocols, measurable outcomes. This wasn't mystical energy work but applied bioelectrical physics - clearing resistance in the body's electrical pathways the same way she'd once debugged network failures. From her home in Portugal, she offers individual sessions and free weekly community healing circles to executives, founders, and high-achievers worldwide who've discovered that sustainable peak performance requires addressing the nervous system at its electrical foundation. Her mission: helping burned-out high-achievers restore their nervous systems when everything else has failed - because burnout isn't a character flaw or psychological weakness, it's a bioelectrical malfunction that can be systematically corrected.

CONNECT WITH JOHANNA:

Website: https://johanna.life

YouTube: https://www.youtube.com/@JohannaFarrimond

LinkedIn: https://www.linkedin.com/in/johannafarrimond/

X: https://x.com/jjfarrimond

The first time I paused in the afternoon to reset,
I was amazed at how I could end the day without
feeling completely drained. I had the energy and
focus to still be present with my partner and then
with a friend at dinner.

~ Garet Free

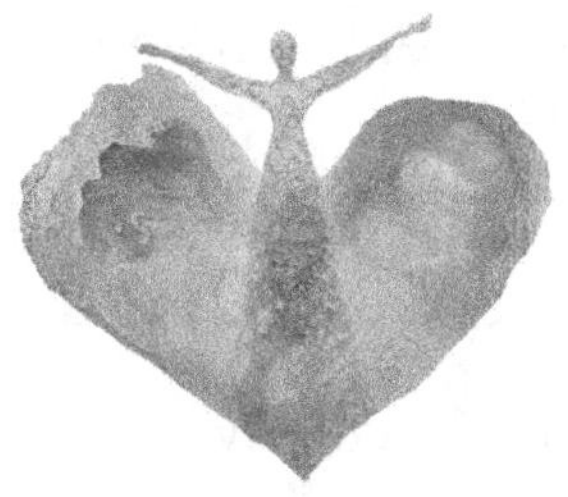

CHAPTER 15

STEADY IS THE NEW STRONG
RECLAIM YOUR FINISH LINE ENERGY

Garet Free

MY STORY

"Maybe if I put a gun in my mouth and pull the trigger, **then** they will fix the healthcare system and the way we treat each other at work."

As these words flowed out of my mouth, my shoulders were tight, my belly was aching, and I couldn't believe I felt this desperate.

It was nearly midnight, the night before my birthday. Work was in pure chaos, my mom was just diagnosed with metastatic breast cancer after two years in remission, and I was raw from a breakup—years of frustrations with life, work, and a system that chews people up boiled over.

My heart pounded out of my chest, and my thoughts raced to the darkest caverns of my mind. Alone on the floor, I sobbed my eyes out, and was shocked at how normal it felt to be this exhausted.

How did I get here?

Building out a plan to end my life was a new low for me. Sure, I had moments in the past where I wondered what my funeral would be like. *What would happen if that bus didn't stop at the stop sign and plowed into me instead?* But seriously contemplating ending my life was a first. I didn't recognize this version of me.

In this moment where anxiety reigned strong, I was desperate for relief and stunned that I was in such a hopeless circumstance.

This was in the messy middle of my healing journey. The part that no one likes to talk about. My journey started a couple of years before the evening when I wanted to pull the trigger for the last time, but this moment was a defining time stamp that I'll never forget. I was moving forward, but this felt like a huge setback. In a moment of such pure hopelessness, where do you turn next?

You rise out of the darkness.

I rallied my close friends, found a therapist, committed to no alcohol for thirty days, and started deepening my inner work. *How do I prevent myself from getting into this level of disrepair again?* Asking for help was rarely on my to-do list. My lifelong mantra was always *I can figure this out.* This time was different. I asked for help and developed a plan because I realized I had to regain control of my life.

The day after my suicidal moment, I was tender—raw. I wanted so badly to celebrate my birthday, but I knew I had to focus on what I would change in the days ahead. Something had to give, and it started with prioritizing myself first.

In the days and weeks that followed, I got back to meditation every morning, set better boundaries with work, started therapy, and leaned into being vulnerable with my friends and family. Not asking for support was no longer an option.

Since I was young, I've been ambitious. I was the yearbook editor in high school and the drum major in band. Just before my 21st birthday, I received my paramedic license and was ready to save the world. That led to the start of my career path, where I poured into others, met them in their moments of crisis, and started to lose myself. My eleven-year career as a paramedic was rewarding yet tough. Sitting with people in their most vulnerable moments, giving them all of my energy, and providing the loving support they needed was my day-to-day experience. I knew people needed support, but I lost myself in strangers. I'm grateful for what I learned, but my unrelenting self-sacrifice was not sustainable.

One evening around 9 p.m., I helped care for a six-week-old baby, still so new to the world. An infection rooted deep in this babe, and he was deathly ill. He lay there in a tangle of lines and alarms while a machine supported his breathing, and his blood pressure was maintained with powerful vasopressor medications. One of those meds was Lēvophed. We have this saying in critical care: "Lēvophed; leave 'em dead." It's morbid, but it speaks to the potent nature of this drug.

Nothing we did worked. It's like his body was saying, "No thanks" to everything. Ninety minutes into a tense resuscitation, I noticed that his mother was sitting in the corner of the trauma bay, all alone, this whole time! She looked terrified and desperate to know if all these hands surrounding her newborn were helping his condition to move in a positive direction.

Stepping over to her, I introduced myself. "Hi I'm Garet. I'm one of the paramedics helping your son." Tears fill my eyes now as I write this story because of the heaviness I felt sitting next to her. Without me saying anything, I saw the grief rising in her eyes. Her puffy and bloodshot eyes were red, but she was all out of tears. She knew things weren't looking good for her son.

With my hand on her back, I absorbed the nervous heat coming from this anxious mom, and tears welled up in my eyes. I told her what we knew, what we didn't, and what we were still trying. I answered the questions she could muster between sniffles and wiping her face, and I had a sinking feeling she'd soon be saying goodbye to the life she recently brought into this world.

She looked over at me, eyes trembling. "What are his chances?"

I had no idea how to respond. It could go either way. "His condition is critical. It's hard to tell, but we're doing our best."

A few hours later, around 2 a.m., after we transferred the child and mom to the ICU, a Code Blue (cardiac arrest) was called. His tiny body couldn't manage any longer, and his time on Earth came to a close.

Those tender moments, usually revolving around the death of a child or loved one, taught me so much, but they also sent my emotions into a downward spiral. Without realizing it, I held on to everything I experienced because I didn't have the tools to release emotions. Throughout my twenties, I did my best, but it wasn't taking me anywhere fast.

Alcohol was my best friend through much of this period. It was so easy to dissociate through blacking out when I had a few days away from work—typically every weekend. It was a vicious pattern that captivated my life for much of my time as a paramedic. I knew something needed to change, and I knew that my time at the bedside had to come to an end.

My first big pivot in life and my career came when I was thirty. I moved to Austin, Texas, and took a new job—changes I desperately craved. I wanted to have a significant impact, and I wanted it now. I told myself that getting into the tech side of healthcare would be so much better. *I'll be happier.*

Getting away from the bedside was necessary, but it didn't fix my "problems." I still drank too much, worked too much, and tried my best to figure out life. I still couldn't release things. Even though things weren't quite as life-and-death, the emotional buildup took its toll.

Does everyone have such a hard time navigating life?

My focus was on work and promotions, but I still struggled with not sleeping well, drinking too much on the weekends, and feeling like I was wandering through life aimlessly—working late into the night, powering through with lots of coffee, and telling myself: *If I keep grinding, it will all work out.* That was my typical day.

I thought if I just hit one more milestone—the promotion, the new house, the relationship—I'd finally feel like I'd made it. But the finish line kept moving. A new race followed every victory I didn't agree to run. That's when I hit rock bottom.

The days and weeks after that fateful night were full of ups and downs. I processed the guilt of slowing down and spent some time in meditation every morning before rushing off to the day ahead. My inner critic was loud, saying things like, "You should be stronger than this."

Once I was back in the groove of meditating every day and focused on getting to the gym, I started to regain some sense of normal.

Fast forward a few years. I navigated the death of my mother, a layoff from a job, and did my best to fight my way through life. Yet I found myself burned out—again.

How did I end up back here? I wasn't drinking; I meditated and took much better care of my body. Yet I still ran on fumes. *You're still pouring out more energy than you're creating!*

The path of healing and repair isn't linear. There will be ups, downs, twists, and turns. It'll all surprise you and teach you the best lessons you never knew you needed, but you have to be open and ready. I've had to accept that rest is productive, and sometimes you need to *just be*—no agenda, no path for dissociating, no end in sight. Just. Be.

Before I knew what regulation was, I felt something inside of me settle when I allowed stillness. Navigating my latest episode of burnout, I found solace in slowing down. It was in these moments that I knew it was time for something completely different.

When I decided to start my own business, I was terrified. I had no idea what I was doing, but I knew I wanted to try something totally different—again. It had been ten years since my last big pivot—*why not pivot again?* I started consulting for startups and growth companies, but I realized my soul was still cranky about doing that work. I needed to get back to my roots as a healer.

My long and winding path to healing and repair could've been cut shorter if I had a trusted guide to keep my focus laser-sharp. I white-knuckled my way through this healing journey with therapy, psychedelics, and reading lots of self-help books, but learned lots of lessons the hard way. As I continued to slow down, I knew that I could make a significant impact on people on a similar journey to mine, so I launched my peak performance and psychedelic therapy practice. Within a year, I wrote a book, started accepting clients, and finally found the alignment I never knew was possible.

Now, mornings start with a ritual that includes morning pages (thank you, Julia Cameron), meditation, pulling three tarot cards, reading, writing, working out (lifting weights four days, yoga two days a week), a shower, and breakfast. I used to get up just in time to throw myself together before my first meeting, and now my day starts by slowing down to care for my needs first.

The steadier I am, especially with caring for myself, the stronger I am in my relationships and my business. For a long time, I wondered why they don't teach us this in school, but I'm happy to have arrived at this moment of clarity today, prioritizing my needs before anything else.

Along the way, I've constantly been challenged with an energy slump in the afternoons. Going strong all day, and then the 2 or 3 p.m. drain comes along. As I continued my healing path, I learned that a regulated and expanded nervous system is critical for success. I started to wonder if I was slipping into dysregulation in the afternoons after sitting at a computer and being in meetings all day, so I blocked off time for an afternoon ritual similar to my morning ritual.

Slowing down isn't just for the mornings. You can also prioritize your needs in the afternoon and evening. Your body has to feel safe before your mind can follow, and the clutter from the day can easily catch up to you in the afternoons. Realizing this became the foundation for a practice I use daily—an afternoon check-in that keeps me steady, even through life's chaos.

FINISHING THE DAY STRONG

You probably don't need *one more thing* on your calendar, but these 30 minutes will give you the space to be more present, clear, and focused for the rest of your day. Powering through those afternoons where everything seems like it's piling up on you doesn't have to weigh you down. You can finish strong with additional energy to show up for yourself, your family, and your friends in the evenings.

The first time I paused in the afternoon to reset, I was amazed at how I could end the day without feeling completely drained. I had the energy and focus to still be present with my partner and then with a friend at dinner. Being present is super important to me, and this ritual helped to bring my presence into greater focus for the remainder of the day.

The weight of irritability, the stiff hips from sitting at a desk all day, and the brain fog from a hectic calendar can be a thing of the past if you choose to prioritize yourself across the day. Even steady leaders fade at 2:30 p.m. I did. Emails stack up, your shoulders start to gather tension, your presence leaks into the ethers. A simple afternoon ritual changed my evenings, my relationships, and my sleep.

THE TOOL

THE AFTERNOON RITUAL

Here's your step-by-step guide, and I can't wait to hear about your experience once you implement this practice.

1. **Block your calendar**

   - Stop reading this book and put a 30-minute block on your calendar around 2 p.m. or 3 p.m.

   - Call it "Afternoon Ritual."

   - Set a reminder notification, and have it repeat daily.

   Put the book down now and go to your calendar.

   Got it done? Great!

   This time is now sacred. You can move it around based on your calendar's needs, but don't delete it or schedule over it.

   Your needs matter before anything else. Remember, you can't pour from an empty cup.

2. For your body - 15 minutes

It's so easy for us to get disconnected from our bodies throughout the day, so the first step is to move.

- Take a walk outside without your phone.

- Touch your toes.

- Stretch.

- Do jumping jacks.

- Body weight squats.

- Dance.

- Shake your body.

- Feel the sun on your face.

Spend fifteen minutes getting into your body.

3. For your mind - 5 minutes

Have a snack. An apple, an orange, an avocado, or a couple of dates. Maybe even some jerky or a handful of nuts. Give your brain the fuel it needs to function.

Enjoy the crunch.

4. For your soul - 5 minutes

Just be.

- Meditate.

- Breathe.

- Lie on the floor

- Write a page in your journal.

  I like to rotate through whatever feels good in the moment. Set a timer for five minutes and go inward.

A couple of my favorite breathing exercises include:

Box breathing: 4-second inhale through your nose, hold for four seconds, 4-second exhale out of your mouth, hold for four seconds, repeat.

4, 7, 8: Inhale through your nose for four seconds, hold for seven seconds, exhale out of your mouth for eight seconds, repeat.

These breathing patterns help to wake up your vagus nerve and bring you back to a sense of calm. Five minutes is all you need.

5. Transition - 5 minutes

Now, get back to your day. Smile. Be grateful you spent this time nurturing yourself, and plan the two to three things that will make the rest of the day a success once you complete them.

If there's anything that's lingering, something that you feel still needs to be shaken off, scream into a pillow. It works wonders.

Thank you

As a token of gratitude for joining me on this ride, I have two things for you:

- Go to https://www.garetfree.com/UG6 to access extra resources for readers of this book. There are videos for guided breath-work and meditations, a guide to psychedelic therapy, and a tracker to help you note the impact of your afternoon ritual on your overall life.

- I'd love to hear from you. When you implement this, please email me and let me know how this practice impacted your life. garet@theresilienceedit.com.

Steady isn't boring, it's brave. Build the habits that hold you when life surges, and your finish line energy won't be a sprint; it'll be your baseline. Start this afternoon. Your future self will feel the difference tonight.

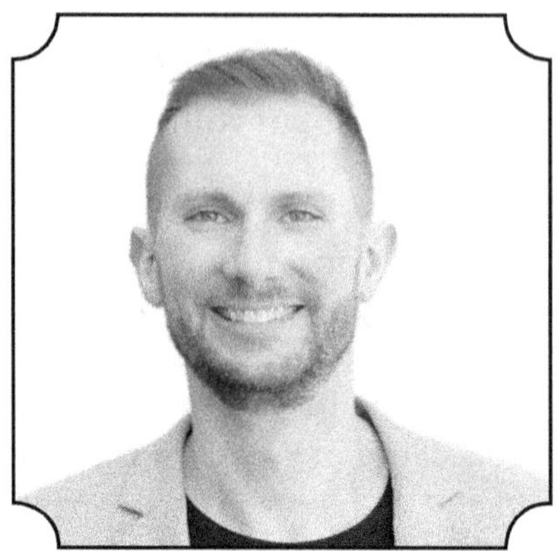

Garet Free is a Peak Performance Coach and Psychedelic Guide who helps entrepreneurs, clinicians, and creatives bridge science and soul to move from survival to sovereignty. Through his healing practice, the resilience edit, and his bestselling book *The Imposter Within,* Garet guides clients to release self-doubt, understand their inner critic, and embody confidence, clarity, and peace.

Before founding the resilience edit, Garet spent more than two decades in healthcare—as a paramedic, consultant, and technology executive—leading teams and building systems designed to help others heal. But after years of outward success paired with inner exhaustion and self-betrayal, he hit a breaking point that forced him to turn inward. His personal journey through addiction, depression, and near-suicidal despair became the catalyst for deep self-healing and the foundation of the work he does today.

Now, Garet blends neuroscience, somatic practices, and psychedelic therapy to help others remember who they are beneath their patterns of performance and perfectionism. His clients learn to regulate their nervous systems, reclaim their power, and create sustainable change from the inside out.

Based in Chicago, Garet is most at home in nature—whether hiking, traveling, or spending slow mornings by the water. He finds restoration in yoga, lifting weights, reading, and losing himself in good house music.

To learn more about Garet's work, connect with him below!

CONNECT WITH GARET:

Website: https://www.garetfree.com

Instagram: https://www.instagram.com/garetfree

Medium: https://medium.com/@garetfree

LinkedIn: https://www.linkedin.com/in/garetfree/

Bluesky: https://bsky.app/profile/garetfree.bsky.social

Buy The Imposter Within: https://a.co/d/el9UZPG

Balancing the nervous system doesn't necessarily mean that your sympathetic nervous system (fight, flight, or freeze) is always balanced with the parasympathetic nervous system (rest, restore). It's considered balanced when the transition between the two is smooth and regular.

~ Michele Silva-Dockery

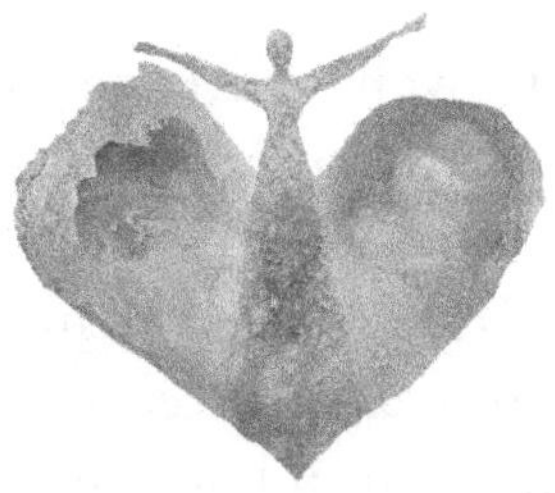

CHAPTER 16

BALANCED BODY, BALANCED LIFE
SIMPLE VAGUS NERVE PRACTICES FOR PERSONAL HEALING

Michele Silva-Dockery

RMT, CECP, CBCP2, CBCP3

MY STORY

Balancing your nervous system can transform your life.

"Sweetheart, I don't have great news." He paused for what seemed like an eternity. "I have cancer. Aggressive prostate cancer." *The C word. Not my soulmate, that can't be!*

Just moments before, my heart felt warm and filled with gratitude for my beloved trees surrounding me. I sat on our beautiful deck thinking about my newfound freedom after retiring from twenty years of teaching. My body tingled with excitement about the life ahead! Dan coming out on the deck interrupted those thoughts. I immediately felt the energy shift. Then came those words. My chest tightened, and my heart sank. Fear and dread replaced joy and gratitude in the pit of my stomach.

That moment shook my world and started me on the path of energy healing—an entirely new chapter. Reiki was the first modality to enter my life. Little did I know the transformative effect it would have on me.

The years 2018-2019 were some of the most challenging of my life. I quickly saw that taking early retirement at age fifty-seven was a blessing and no coincidence.

Dan's cancer treatment involved five weeks of radiation. Then came radioactive implant surgery. Suddenly, the medical world was a constant part of our lives. *We will overcome this together. We have to!* But there was even more to overcome. During his treatment, we lost three friends who were too young. Both my sons experienced separate traumatic events that were tough for this mom's heart to endure. My mother, too, slipped further into dementia.

I have to find a way to get my joy back.

"When was the last time you gave yourself Reiki?" A friend of mine, a Reiki Master, knew what I was going through. We called each other regularly to check in. I couldn't remember the last time I did any self-Reiki since learning the beautiful modality. When I took my first Reiki class, I didn't feel much at first, but then, subtle shifts happened. My intuition opened, and I became more sensitive to the energy around me. My hands and my heart warmed when Reiki energy flowed through. "Thank you, my friend!" *I needed this reminder. It's easy to forget to practice self-care during overwhelming times. I'll start back tomorrow!*

Then came the dreaded Lupron shots. To prevent prostate cancer from spreading, doctors gradually eliminate all testosterone. The night before Dan's first shot, my heart broke into little pieces. After his intense workout in the basement, I heard him play a song we both loved—a song of deep sadness and loss, as well as of hope and longing. Tears rolled down my cheek. I felt helpless. *For the first time since we met, I don't know how to comfort him. What can I do? My body aches—I sense his despair.*

He was barely 60 years old, full of life, actively pursuing his hobbies, and supervising over 200 staff at his job; he knew that could change, perhaps forever. The effects of the Lupron treatment were harsh on both of us. Over the course of ten months, Dan's resilience and endurance declined, and the hormonal changes were exhausting.

I want my Dan back. I want to learn everything I can to help him heal!

As Dan's journey continued, I delved deeper into learning Reiki and explored additional tools for managing stress and overwhelm. I gave Dan Reiki sessions and practiced as often as I could with him, friends, and family, even several animal companions! Receiving feedback and validation built my confidence. I knew that when life became more manageable, I'd pursue the Reiki Master level.

Throughout my husband's battle with cancer, my elderly mother became less independent and more confused. Dementia took over the mom I knew. I was heartbroken. My heart ached for the witty, talented, nature-loving person she once was. I missed our long walks in the park. I longed for her to remember like she used to. I grieved—even though she was still alive.

Full-time caregiving became a necessity. Being her only child, I was thrown into that role.

"Try to smile when you wake up in the morning, even if it's the last thing you want to do. It will shift your energy. There is research to back that up." *Smile? How can I do that when I dread the day?* But I trusted Sandra completely and tried it as often as I could. I experienced a slight shift. I loved how simple it was.

I was blessed to work with Sandra, a life coach, for several months. She opened my eyes to many tools available to help with stress, anxiety, overwhelm, and trauma. She had intuitive wisdom. I wanted that too. New worlds opened up to me. I felt hopeful for the first time in a long time. I woke up in the mornings feeling lighter and optimistic, rather than the familiar dread. I didn't always have to force a smile in the morning.

I knew in my heart that Dan would make it. I felt a tingling sensation throughout my body, confirming my belief. Dan has now been cancer-free for over five years, with his Lupron experience a distant memory! I also knew my sons would overcome their challenges and come out stronger, which they eventually did.

When I juggled supporting Dan, my family, and caring for my mom, I constantly felt overwhelmed. It took a toll on my body. My chest often felt like bricks pressed on it. Deep breaths became difficult. My body ached. Self-care and self-Reiki seemed like distant dreams. I needed quick tools that worked fast and could be used anywhere. Caregivers often don't have time to use techniques to help them de-stress. Finding time to sit and meditate, journal, or practice breathwork? It can feel overwhelming.

While exploring ways to cope, I discovered literature on the vagus nerve and the many benefits of keeping it balanced. *That's it! That's what I need. This could also help Dan!*

Discovering this felt like the next piece of the puzzle—exactly what was needed and possibly what could help Dan, I found small pockets of time to read books and take courses on the topic. Almost immediately, I started applying some suggested protocols to myself, like bracing for unpredictable situations during elevator rides to my mother's apartment. Just taking a few minutes for myself on the way up made a huge difference in how I handled her extreme moods.

My mother fell more frequently. Eventually, she was rushed to the emergency room. She could no longer live on her own. After a frantic search for a rehab—and eventually, a nursing home I felt comfortable with—she was accepted and we made plans for her move. I visited her every day in the hospital, doing my best to comfort and help her with her confusion.

The day I was supposed to help her move into her new place, all rehabs, assisted living facilities, and nursing homes shut down because of the pandemic. When I heard this, my throat tightened and I felt numb. *How can she go through this alone?* My last hospital visit was the final time I saw her alive in person.

Several months later, my mother passed peacefully one morning with a caring hospice nurse by her side. The COVID-19 pandemic marked a new chapter in my personal healing. I used this time to grieve deeply, process my emotions, and reflect on my recent experiences. Throughout my life, I've always viewed challenges as learning opportunities. This period helped me become a Reiki master teacher, incorporate Reiki into my daily life, and earn certifications in additional healing modalities. Eventually, I founded my first company at age 64, a step that felt deeply aligned and revealed a sense of purpose I longed for during my later years of teaching. Becoming an energy healer felt incredibly rewarding—almost like an unexpected miracle.

My heart feels whole, and joy flows throughout my body. Surrounded by my beloved trees with their stunning fall colors, I sit peacefully on the deck. I'm grateful for the opportunity to help others transform their lives. Sharing Reiki with others truly puts me in my happy place. I wake up eager to begin the day. I love what I do. What could be better than helping others release energy blocks that keep them from living their lives to the fullest?

What I share in the next section is a list of quick ways to relieve stress, anxiety, overwhelm, or all of the above. I used these techniques when I was in the middle of feeling like my world was falling apart. I needed tools I could use anywhere without seeming weird, tools that worked fast.

Learning to regulate my nervous system changed my life.

THE TOOL

Balancing the nervous system doesn't necessarily mean that your sympathetic nervous system (fight, flight, or freeze) is always balanced with the parasympathetic nervous system (rest, restore). It's considered balanced when the transition between the two is smooth and regular.

The vagus nerve, often called the "wandering nerve," is one of the most vital pathways connecting the brain to the body. It runs from the brainstem (at the base of the skull) through the neck, chest, and abdomen, touching nearly every major organ along its path. As the primary nerve of the parasympathetic nervous system, it helps regulate heart rate, digestion, immune response, and relaxation. When it's balanced and working correctly, the vagus nerve promotes a calm mind, stable emotions, a strong immune system, and overall well-being. Many self-healing practices—such as deep breathing, humming, meditation, energy healing, and gentle movement—stimulate and tone the vagus nerve, helping the body shift from stress to calm.

- **Conscious breathing.** There are many effective techniques, like "box breathing," and others that involve counting both the inhale and exhale. I love breathwork and all the ways to use conscious breath. It's one of the best ways to reset and calm the nervous system. It's also an essential part of vagus nerve protocols.

My husband, along with some clients, gets distracted by counting. My advice in this case is to keep it simple: exhale longer than you inhale. This signals your nervous system that you're safe. I find it easy to remember when I feel anxiety coming on. When I notice myself doing "chest breathing," I make sure I exhale longer so I don't trigger my sympathetic nervous system.

- **Holding your forehead.** You may have noticed that people often place their hands on their foreheads when they're surprised or shocked. We instinctively know about self-healing tools without realizing it. When feeling anxious or stressed, rest your hand on your forehead. It's easy to do anywhere and is hardly noticeable by others. The amount of pressure can vary depending on what feels right for you. Sometimes I prefer a gentle touch; other times, I need more pressure. Listen to your body and trust its cues. Doing this signals your sympathetic system to slow down. It works quickly. The forehead involves the cranial nerve. To activate the vagus nerve, you can hold your forehead with one hand and the base of your skull with the other. Deep breathing or humming will further stimulate it, resulting in more effective outcomes. Do this for a few minutes at a time.

- **Finger behind the earlobe.** Place your middle finger behind the soft part of each earlobe, with your other fingers cupping your cheeks and throat. No need to use pressure, just a soft touch. The insides of your wrists will touch at the base of your throat. Take deep belly breaths. Humming is even better if you're alone. This is an excellent way to regulate your vagus nerve daily. It works quickly, so three to five minutes can be enough.

As I mentioned earlier, the vagus nerve begins at the brainstem. It then loops around the ears, down the throat, and to all the organs in the body. When you place a finger behind your earlobe, you're touching a gateway to the vagus nerve. Doing this with conscious breathing, especially humming or toning, can help stimulate and tone your vagus nerve. I notice a significant difference in stress relief when I do this every day.

- **Scanning for shapes or colors.** This method worked really well for me a few months ago when I was overwhelmed and panicked. Tears were flowing, my heart was pounding, and taking deep breaths felt difficult. I stood in our family room and chose a color that looked calming to me. I slowly scanned the room for that color, noticing what I saw. Scan each wall, the ceiling, the floor, windows, and doors (if any), at a slow, steady pace. If you still feel anxious, pick a shape and scan the room again. Do this as long as needed. Be sure to do this slowly, with a sense of curiosity. This helps signal safety and can help your nervous system regain balance.

- **Hands on the heart and naval.** When I feel my heart beating fast or anxiety coming on, I place one hand on my heart and the other on my belly button. I do this especially early in the morning while I lie in bed and try to go back to sleep. The warmth and gentle pressure feel deeply comforting. Touching the naval area can help calm the body's stress response and support vagal regulation through mindful breathing and connection.

- **Micro-moments.** No matter how busy our days are, we can find a few minutes (micro-moments) throughout the day to sit down and close our eyes (or have a soft gaze). Some of those minutes can even be during a bathroom break! Taking tiny, quiet moments to do absolutely nothing can reset our nervous system. By "absolutely nothing," I mean not even thinking about the breath, trying to meditate, or anything else besides being in stillness. If that feels too difficult at first and your mind is constantly chattering, then focus on your breath. Start with one micro-moment for a few days. Then increase to two, and eventually three. Consider each moment a reset for your system. It will do wonders.

- **Journaling.** Choose one of the quotes below and write down the emotions you're feeling. Pour everything onto paper (or electronically) without overthinking what you're writing. If unpleasant emotions arise, allow yourself to feel them and keep writing. You might be surprised by what a quote sparks in you. Writing is almost always healing. Optional: If one of the quotes resonates with you, keep it visible throughout your day and repeat it three or more times. Say it as if it's already true, and really feel the emotions it stirs.

Quotes:

"I am doing my best, and that is enough."

"I am allowed to take time for myself."

"I am worthy of love and respect."

"I am deserving of care and compassion."

"I release the need to be perfect."

Choose what resonates with you. Explore more vagus nerve protocols that appeal to you—there are so many! Trust that whatever stress you're going through, it CAN—and it WILL—improve. Self-help tools are simply that: self-help that empowers you to take control.

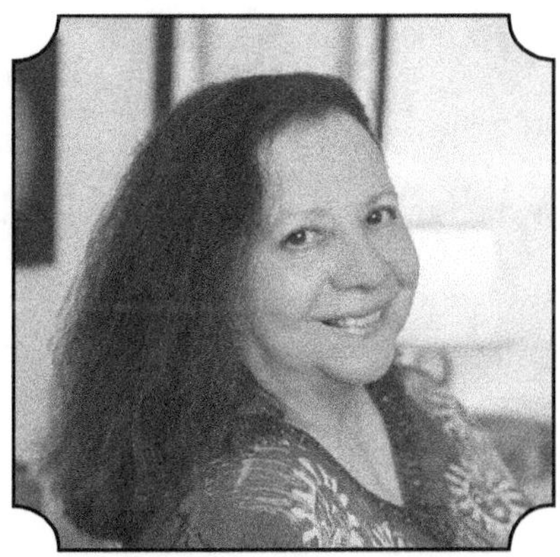

Michele Silva-Dockery is a Reiki Master Teacher, Emotion Code, Body Code, and Belief Code Practitioner, and the founder of Caring Onward, a heart-centered practice dedicated to helping individuals release emotional and energetic imbalances that limit their well-being. Drawing on her background as a mathematics educator for over thirty years and her lifelong curiosity about the connection between mind, body, and spirit, Michele combines grounded wisdom with intuitive insight in her work.

Through her sessions and classes, Michele helps clients release trapped emotions, identify limiting beliefs, and restore energetic balance—enabling the body's natural healing. Her clients often say they feel lighter, more peaceful, and better able to handle life's challenges. Some say their lives have been transformed.

Michele's personal journey with energy healing strengthened her belief that true healing involves not just the physical but also the emotional, mental, and spiritual aspects of life. She now dedicates her work to helping others with tools for self-healing so they can move forward with renewed confidence and purpose.

In addition to private sessions, Michele teaches Usui Reiki Levels 1 through 3, both online and in person. She offers courses designed to help students connect deeply with Reiki as both a healing art and a spiritual journey. Her passion is in helping others realize that healing isn't about fixing what's broken—it's about remembering who we truly are beneath the layers of stress, fear, and pain.

CONNECT WITH MICHELE:

Website: https://caringonward.com

Instagram: https://www.instagram.com/caringonward/

Facebook: https://www.facebook.com/profile.php?id=61561295146370

LinkedIn:
https://www.linkedin.com/in/michele-silva-dockery-b8a756123/

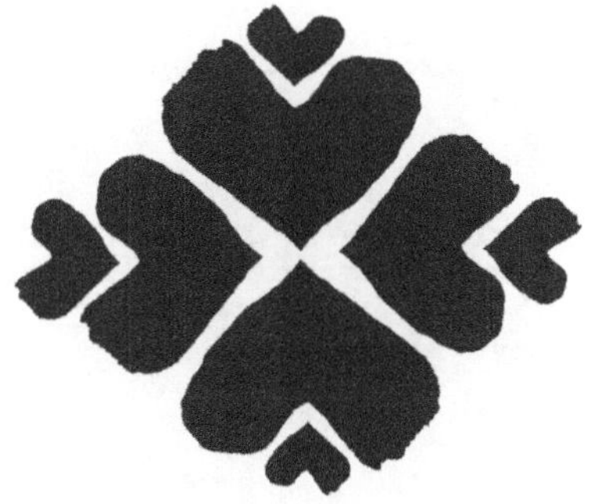

EXPERIENCING GRIEF

Even though death has changed our relationship, it has not ended our connection. The love I feel remains within me. I carry you with me, always.

~ Kelly Daugherty

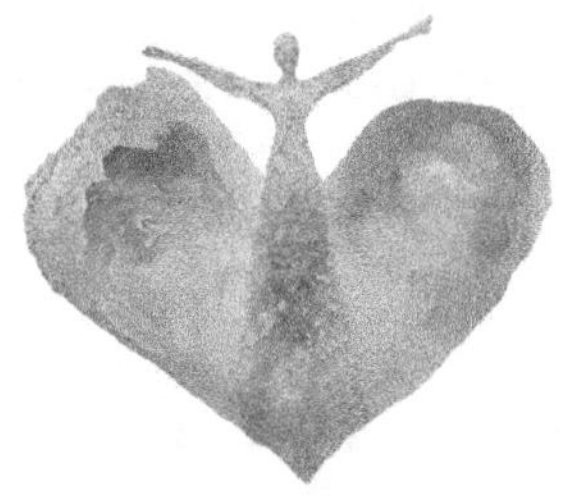

CHAPTER 17

CELEBRATE THEIR LIFE
FOCUSING ON GRATITUDE, CONNECTION, AND WHAT STILL REMAINS

Kelly Daugherty

LCSW-R, FT, BCC

MY STORY

She's missed out on so much.

It's not fair.

She never got to meet her grandchildren.

She never got to meet my husband.

These were the thoughts that constantly ran through my mind for many years. Since my mom died, I've found myself grieving her in different ways ever since. Each milestone and celebration, and every moment I needed her hug or her advice, felt like another loss. I focused on everything my mom missed and all the things I didn't get to do with her.

My mom died when I was 14 years old from breast cancer, and that loss shaped my life and who I am today. I became a grief counselor because of it, yet I still struggled to feel genuinely connected to her and focus on what **I did** get to do with her.

When I met my husband, it had been almost 20 years since my mom died, but I was still caught in that same struggle, focusing on what she missed instead of what remained. My husband noticed it, "Why don't you write a letter to her?"

This is something I've done many times before, probably 50 times. But I trusted him and his instincts, so I did it.

As I wrote, I told her what I missed about her, but more importantly, what I learned from her while she was here, and what I learned through her death and my own grief. I began to move away from the pain I held and into something new: gratitude. Something shifted for me when I wrote that letter.

I went from focusing on what I lost to focusing on what I still had. Gratitude took shape for the lessons my mom taught me, the memories we shared, and the ways she shaped who I am through both her life and her death. My grief didn't disappear, but it evolved. I didn't just see what was missing anymore; I finally recognized all that remained. That letter didn't bring her back, but it changed how I experienced my grief.

I began to notice the ways she continued to influence my life, and I finally saw that love and gratitude could coexist with grief. Over time, that perspective deepened. I found new ways to remember her, celebrating her birthday and the anniversary of her death by focusing on her life and our connection. As I did these things, I felt relief, gratitude, and more at peace.

That experience also shaped how I support others in their grief. I learned to celebrate my mom's life, and I hope others can find that same shift of honoring the person who died by celebrating their life. This allows people to shift their focus from the death and what is lost to honoring their loved ones not by letting go, but by recognizing the love, lessons, and connection that remain. It's about embracing grief and remembrance, allowing people to move forward without leaving their loved ones behind.

Celebrating Their Life isn't about forgetting; it's about carrying their presence forward in a meaningful way. While death changes everything, it doesn't erase the bond and connection we share with those who've died.

As I write this now, it's been almost a year since my dad died. I find myself back in early grief again, challenged to apply the same perspective I found with my mom. My dad was 90 when he died. Many people said, "He had a great life," but his death still came as a shock. We had just celebrated his 90th birthday, and aside from some minor aches and pains, he appeared to be in good health. Three months later, he was diagnosed with metastatic prostate cancer, and within four months, I held his hand as he took his final breaths in a hospice facility.

As I navigate this loss, I remind myself: *Focus on the gratitude that you had Dad for 45 years.* Would I have wanted more time? Of course. It never would've been long enough. But we made incredible memories together.

After my mom died, my dad and I had to build our relationship. Before then, my mom was the caretaker; she took care of all of us, including him. My dad was the provider, working long hours while she managed our daily lives. As a teenager, I was interviewed for a local cable news show about my experience as a grieving teen. During this segment, my dad was interviewed over the phone and stated, "It seemed that there were two different families. I was one of them; my wife and daughters were the other family. I was working most of the time trying to put my two daughters through college, and as a consequence, I didn't have much time to spend with my children." And that was true, my sisters and I were not close to my dad. My dad was actively drinking for many years, and this also caused a significant strain on our relationship with him and made him more unavailable to us when he was home.

After my mom's death, we had to find a new way to survive without her, and it wasn't easy. We struggled to figure out what our relationship would look like. My sisters moved out of our family home shortly after my mom's death, which meant it was just me and my dad. My dad's drinking worsened, and the arguing between the two of us was daily. Things weren't good between us at home. I felt so alone in my grief and cried myself to sleep most nights, longing for my mom and the relationship I had with her. I was angry at my dad. I was angry at God. *Why did God take my mom?*

I recall during several heated arguments with my dad saying, "I wish you had died instead of Mom!" and I meant that at that time. As things continued to decline at home with my dad, I made a desperate attempt to make things change. On a cold winter day in January, approximately six months after my mom died, I wrote my dad a letter threatening to run away if he didn't stop drinking. I was fifteen, heartbroken over my mom's death, and desperate for things to change; I was determined to run away if things didn't change.

He stood in the doorway of my bedroom after reading the letter and said, "I don't have a problem with drinking alcohol, but I'll stop." Those first months of his sobriety without any intervention for his alcoholism were rough, really rough, with lots of screaming matches and poor communication. We attended family therapy during that time, and I still have deep appreciation and respect for how our psychologist, Margaret, helped us navigate those intense and really difficult sessions.

Two years into my dad's sobriety, our close family friend and neighbor invited him to Alcoholics Anonymous (AA), and he went. That invitation changed the course of his life and our relationship. By the time he died, he was sober for almost thirty years and a member of AA for nearly twenty-eight.

In the years that followed, we had many honest conversations. He made amends to me for his actions when he was drinking and how it impacted our lives. We talked about how difficult those years were with his drinking, his behavior, and how it impacted us all. In time, we found understanding.

The night before he died, I told him, "Dad, if anyone has taught me that people are capable of change, it's you. I'm so proud of you for getting sober all those years ago and for the man you became. You have taught me people can change." Was my dad perfect? No, not at all. But none of us are. And while there were things he still struggled with even at ninety, he made tremendous progress in his life. I'm proud of the man he became.

Focusing on gratitude doesn't mean I forget my dad, and it doesn't mean I don't grieve. Grief and gratitude can coexist. That's the beauty of grief: we can miss them deeply while also being grateful for all they gave us. I'm finding my way to celebrate my dad's life as I grieve for him.

Two months after my dad died, my sisters and I traveled to Florida to have a service for his friends and his AA community. His funeral was held on Long Island, where we grew up, and where he wanted to be buried with our mom, but we knew we needed to do something in Florida, where he had lived since 1997.

Following the Florida church service, we gathered with his AA community and heard stories about our dad, the man they knew, the man who supported others in their recovery. I talked at this gathering, shared my story of my relationship with my dad, and thanked the AA community. "Thank you for giving me the chance to have a relationship with my dad. I genuinely believe that without my dad becoming sober, I would've never grown to love and appreciate him, and we would've never had the connection we had." At the end of the gathering, my sister said, "The funeral was for us; this was for dad." She was right; it was about our dad, his legacy, and it was a beautiful way to honor him and celebrate his life. I'm so grateful we did that.

Today, I specialize in grief and loss. Through my grief counseling practice, I support grieving individuals, and with the Center for Informed Grief, I train therapists and school professionals to be truly grief-informed. I've written books, developed grief groups and life-changing retreats, and created spaces for thousands of grieving people to acknowledge their loss without the pressure to "move on." My work focuses on helping people integrate grief into their lives and maintain a connection to their loved ones, and that's how I find meaning in my grief.

That moment of writing to my mom shifted everything, including how I grieve for my dad and how I show up to support others in their grief experience. It helped me see that while death changes our relationship, it doesn't end it. Gratitude continues to be my way to stay connected to both my parents, to shift my focus from what was lost, but to what remains. Every time I speak my parents' names, share their stories, or help someone else do the same, I'm reminded of my continued connection to them, and I can truly celebrate their lives.

The Tool

This tool is to help you shift your mindset from loss to celebrating the lives of those you loved who've died. Everyone's grief is different. Every relationship is unique. These prompts are meant to help you discover what feels right for you in your grief and to find meaningful ways to celebrate your loved one's life.

Here are some of the ways I do this in my own life:

I make my mom's chocolate every Christmas season with friends, using the molds we used together when I was a child. I wear her Christmas pins during the holidays and her jewelry year-round. I wear jewelry my dad gave me. I have pictures of both my parents in my home and office, and I display my dad's Navy flag as a reminder of him.

I talk to them out loud. I talk about them, share memories, and use their names. These may sound like small things, but they truly make a difference. They help shift my focus from what's missing to what remains: love, connection, and the gratitude for all I gained from them.

One of my clients once told me, "I keep going because I want to be the storyteller of my loved one's life." She wants to keep saying their names, keep talking about them, and keep sharing who they were. That, to me, is what it's all about: continuing their story and celebrating their life.

Here are some prompts to help you start thinking about how to celebrate your loved one's life. This exercise is designed to help you reconnect with moments that bring warmth, gratitude, and a sense of connection to the person who died. It's about intentionally shifting your focus toward what remains: the love, memories, and lessons that continue to live within you.

STEP 1: MEMORY PROMPTS

Begin by jotting down a few memories that evoke a sense of comfort, gratitude, or closeness. These don't have to be major moments. Often, it's the small, ordinary memories that bring the strongest connection.

Use these prompts to get started:

- A moment that still makes me smile when I think of them is. . .

- One thing they taught me that I still carry with me is. . .

- When I picture them at peace, I see them. . .

- A sound, smell, or song that instantly brings them to mind is. . .

- I feel closest to them when I. . .

- Something they used to say or do that I find myself repeating is. . .

Take a few minutes to write freely. Let the memories surface without judging or filtering them.

STEP 2: CELEBRATE THEIR LIFE: HEART CONNECTION MEDITATION

During this meditation, I'll ask you to place your hand over your heart and breathe a little differently than you're used to, exhaling more than you inhale. It's important to follow these directions; they help create heart coherence, a state where your heart, mind, emotions, and body work together in a calmer, more connected manner. Our hearts often feel a deeper bond with our loved ones than our minds do, and this practice helps you connect to that space within you.

If you would prefer to listen to this meditation, visit:

https://www.kellydaugherty.com/books

Take a moment to find a comfortable position.

Let your body settle, allowing your shoulders to drop, and relax your jaw.

When you're ready, bring one or both hands to your heart.

Feel your hand resting there, and notice your heart beating beneath it.

Take a slow, steady breath in and as you exhale, breathe out a little more than you took in.

There's no need to count, but if it feels right, breathe in for a count of four and exhale for a count of six or whatever feels natural to you.

Imagine your breath flowing in and out of your heart.

Lean into the rhythm of your breath, the gentle rise and fall.

With each exhale, allow yourself to relax a little more.

With every cycle of your breath, feel that space in your heart where your loved one continues to live within you.

As you continue to breathe in and out of your heart, notice your body beginning to relax.

Notice the stillness.

You're connecting to the part of yourself that remembers, the place where your love for your loved one still lives inside of you.

Now, bring to mind a memory of your loved one that brings warmth, comfort, or gratitude.

It doesn't have to be a big moment. Maybe it's a shared laugh, a look, a small gesture, a positive memory, or something that reminds you of being close.

Let that memory come to you; there's no right or wrong.

Let that memory fill your awareness—see it, feel it, hear it. Notice the emotions that memory stirs within you.

As you continue breathing through your heart, let yourself feel that connection.

Let the love, appreciation, and gratitude from that moment expand within you.

With each breath, imagine that connection growing, spreading from your heart through your chest, down your arms, and throughout your entire body.

Stay here for a few breaths. Continue exhaling longer than you inhale, and breathe through your heart.

Connected to gratitude.

Connected to love.

Now, as you rest in this feeling, quietly say to yourself:

"Even though death has changed our relationship, it has not ended our connection."

"The love I feel remains within me."

"I carry you with me, always."

Take one final deep breath in through your heart and out through your heart.

Before moving on, ask yourself: *What is one small thing I can do today to celebrate their life?*

Maybe it's speaking their name, sharing a story, lighting a candle, or carrying forward something they taught you.

Each act of remembrance is a way to celebrate their life and a reminder that love doesn't end. It continues in you.

When you feel ready, gently open your eyes and return to the present moment.

STEP 3: ACTIONABLE STEPS

Now that you have listened to the meditation, take a few minutes to identify one small, tangible thing you can do to celebrate your loved one's life. It doesn't have to be big or elaborate. Sometimes the smallest gestures are the most meaningful.

Some ideas may include:

- Saying their name out loud or sharing a story about them.

- Cooking their favorite meal or creating a cookbook with their best recipes.

- Make a playlist of your loved one's favorite songs.

- Light a candle, wear something that connects you to them, or visit a special place.

- Engaging in a hobby that your loved one enjoyed.

- Continue a tradition they loved.

- Finding a ritual that makes hard days feel more peaceful.

- Do something they valued, such as an act of kindness, volunteering, or helping someone in need.

Once you've identified what feels meaningful, do it with intention and love.

After you do something to celebrate their life, take a moment to reflect and answer these questions:

- What was it like to do this?

- What emotions came up for me?

- How did it feel to celebrate their life?

Celebrating Their Life helps keep their memory alive and the connection we shared with them. Although death changes everything, the love and connection you shared with them always remain.

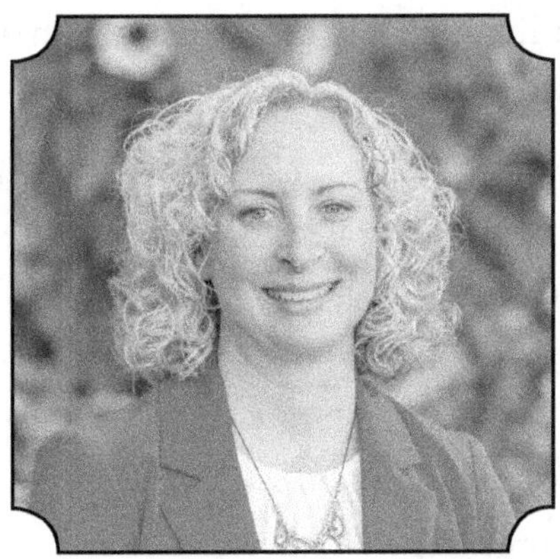

Kelly Daugherty is a Licensed Clinical Social Worker, Fellow in Thanatology: Death, Dying, and Bereavement, and Board-Certified Coach with more than twenty-five years of experience supporting grieving individuals and training professionals to become more grief-informed. Based in Malta, New York, she owns Kelly Daugherty, LCSW, PLLC and The Center for Informed Grief, LLC, where she provides counseling, professional trainings, and consultation to schools and organizations seeking to create more grief-informed environments.

Kelly's dedication to this work began after her mother died of breast cancer when she was fourteen years old, a loss that shaped her life and career. Volunteering with a children's bereavement program through hospice became the foundation for what has grown into a lifelong commitment to helping others find meaning after loss.

Through the Center for Informed Grief, Kelly develops and delivers training for therapists, educators, and helping professionals nationwide. Her programs focus on building grief-informed cultures in schools and workplaces through research-based education, practical tools, and actionable strategies.

An accomplished author and educator, Kelly has contributed to *Holistic Mental Health* and *Brave Kids, Volumes 1, 2,* and *3,* and led the collaborative book *The Grief Experience: Tools for Acceptance, Resilience, and Connection.* She is also the co-host of The GRIEF Ladies Podcast, where she and Karyn Arnold share honest conversations and actionable steps from their GRIEF

Framework to help individuals integrate loss into their lives in meaningful ways and move forward with purpose.

When she's not working, Kelly enjoys time with her husband, Kevin, and their Boston Terrier, Benny. She loves spending time with her nieces and nephews, walking and running outdoors, and visiting beaches, zoos, and Disney World.

CONNECT WITH KELLY:

LinkTree: https://linktr.ee/kellydaugherty

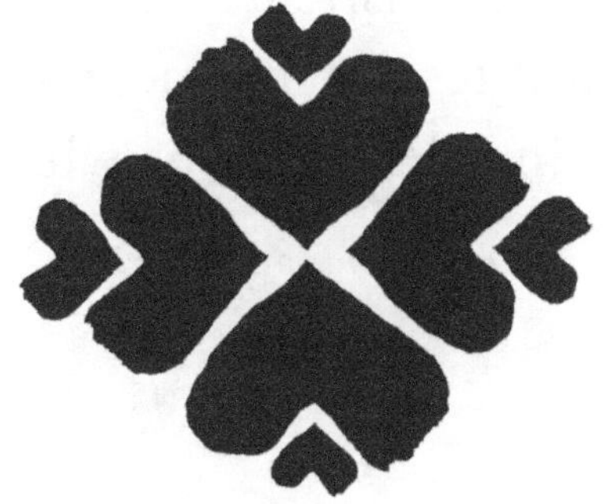

What if the body isn't just an archive of old wounds? What if it's a dynamic, energetic system? Even in grief, it hums with life.

~ Dr. Faith Galliano Desai

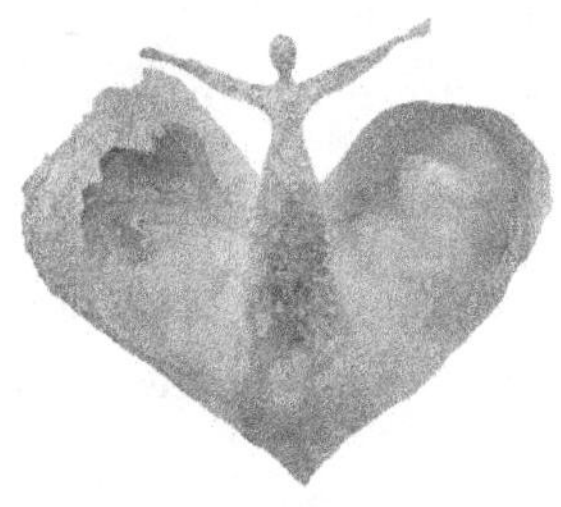

Chapter 18

Living Grief

The F.E.E.L. Method for Moving with Emotion

Dr. Faith Galliano Desai

PSYCHOLOGIST

My Story

Grief doesn't always announce itself with loss. Sometimes, it begins in the middle of life, when everything still looks intact.

I remember the night I rushed my mom to the hospital. She struggled to breathe, her chest rising and falling in shallow gasps. By the time we arrived, she was unconscious. Something in me went still, as if my body already knew life had divided itself into before and after. I stood at her bedside, listening to the machines fill the silence with their steady beeping, doing the work her body couldn't. *Please open your eyes. Please just come back.*

The diagnosis hit like a blunt instrument: end-stage renal failure. "She might have a year or two, but we can't really know," the doctors said.

In the weeks that followed, time lost its edges. Days blurred into hospital corridors and waiting rooms that smelled faintly of disinfectant and coffee. I lived hour by hour, holding my breath between each beep of the monitor, praying she'd open her eyes, dreading she might not.

When she finally stabilized enough to begin dialysis, relief came laced with more dread. Borrowed time, no promise. That uncertainty became the air we breathed.

Hope became its own kind of ache. Each improvement felt like a miracle, and a countdown at the same time.

She lived for seven years—seven years of fragile stability, sudden downturns, and unexpected rallies. Seven years of holding gratitude and grief in the same breath. What I carried home wasn't just a diagnosis; it was the unknowing, the weight of waiting. Every day could be the last, yet every day kept coming.

Grief isn't always a storm. Sometimes, it's the still air before one that never comes. Some mornings, I woke up with relief—others with dread. Gratitude and fear lived side by side, like two hands gripping the same thread.

That's how I learned to live in the in-between, not with answers or certainty, but with breath. I didn't know it then, but this was my initiation into living grief.

I didn't realize my body carried the grief as much as my heart. In those early weeks, I told myself: *You're just tired from hospital runs and sitting beside her bed trying to hold everything together.* But it was more. My chest tightened, my shoulders locked, sleep fractured. I held my breath without meaning to and lived as if exhaling meant surrender.

I called it exhaustion, but it was my body trying to have a conversation I wasn't ready to hear. It told the story long before I had words.

I moved quickly between extremes, numb one moment, flooded the next. Hope, fear, anger, gratitude. They all lived inside me at once. No neat order. Just waves. Just energy.

Living with grief changed how I related to myself. It stripped away illusions of control and forced me to sit with questions I couldn't answer.

It taught me that silence can be heavy, and that the body's instinct to freeze is often just a longing for safety.

What surprised me most wasn't just *this* grief. It stirred up grief I thought I'd already survived. Sitting by my mom's bed, holding my breath, I felt the present's sharpness mingle with old wounds I didn't know I still carried. Every unshed tear, every past loss rose to the surface and blended with this one.

The weight of waiting opened a cracked door inside me. Past and present moved through me together, wave upon wave, leaving me raw and unsure where one ended and the other began.

Even healing can become another way to hide. I know, because I did it. In that rawness, I wasn't always honest with myself. I learned practices I thought helped me regulate, but they often became ways to bypass what I felt. Breathing techniques, affirmations, reframes, I used them as shields, ways to skip over grief instead of moving through it.

I called it "self-regulation," but really, I controlled, repressed, and polished the parts I thought were acceptable. I caught myself rehearsing the "right" way to grieve, waiting for someone to see me, to comfort me.

Then, I began to experience self-regulation differently. Not as calming down or mastering myself, but as a relationship, a conversation between the body and what lives inside it. Sensations weren't problems; they were energy—undirected, urgent, alive, wanting to be welcomed and felt.

Living grief taught me how messy that welcome is. Regulation isn't about feeling calm all the time. It's about being willing to feel everything: anger, joy, rage, grief. They exist all at once.

And when the feelings get too big to hold alone, we sometimes start to reach for witnesses.

At some point, grief stopped being private. It became something I performed just to be seen, measured in the tilt of a head, a sympathetic sigh, a hand on my shoulder. I started mistaking recognition for relief. Living grief can do that. It's so complex, it blurs the line between being witnessed and being known.

I realized I outsourced safety to others' reactions: if they nodded or comforted me, I felt okay; if not, exposed. My safety wasn't mine. It lived in their acceptance. And when safety depends on that, the body never truly rests.

That pushed me up against my freeze response. I hid parts of myself so well, even from me, that when they surfaced, I didn't know what to do. Living grief wasn't only waiting for my mother's decline; it faced pieces of myself I exiled for years, realizing they knocked on the same door.

Everything inside me was noise. Nothing made sense, but everything felt true. What I felt wasn't safety vanishing; it was undirected energy: heat in my chest, pressure behind my eyes, tremor in my hands. Not "grief" here and "anger" there, but current after current with nowhere to go. Not even a feeling I could name, only a tangled, insistent hum moving through me.

That's when something shifted. *If emotions can blur and spill into one another, maybe naming isn't the point. Maybe what matters is movement, the way sensation wants to travel, release, become something else.*

What I experienced wasn't chaos. It was energy asking for form.

I began to see emotions differently, not moods to manage or fix, but currents of energy moving through my nervous system. My grief, anger, and even joy weren't intruders or evidence that I was broken. They were energy—restless, insistent, and alive—asking to move.

When I stopped treating emotions as threats to regulate away and started relating to them as energy, I found space where before there was only overwhelm. I paused without shutting down, listened without drowning, let emotions move through me instead of burying or performing them for acceptance.

In that space, I heard what my body was saying all along.

The body remembers, but not as stories. Trauma isn't an archive of terrible events; it's any moment, big, small, subtle, ordinary, that overwhelms the nervous system's ability to respond and return to safety. These moments live not as narrative but as activation, sensation, energy.

Emotions are chemical and hormonal events. When the brain sends out those signals, you feel them: a racing heart, tight muscles, a sinking in the gut. Left alone, those sensations often pass within about ninety seconds. But when the mind loops, replaying the story, it traps the body's response. That's how emotions get stuck circling, echoing, waiting for movement.

And that's why trauma isn't about categories; it's about overwhelm. Sometimes, it happens in a single instant. Sometimes, it builds quietly, too much for too long, or not enough for too long. These moments live between "good enough" and "safe enough." On the outside, they may look ordinary. Inside, they live as everything.

So, what if the body isn't just an archive of old wounds? What if it's a dynamic, energetic system? Even in grief, it hums with life.

It breathes, responds, creates. Yes, it carries echoes of what's unresolved, but it also pulses with joy, sparks with curiosity, dances with possibilities.

The body speaks in physics: waves of sensation, patterns of tension and release, rhythms of contraction and expansion. Every emotion has its signature: joy expands, fear tightens, shame curls in, anger pushes out. These aren't random; they're the nervous system's choreography, responding to what's happening inside and around us.

When anxiety ripples through your chest or shame settles in your gut, these aren't abstract feelings. They're energy in motion, tangible, somatic, as real as a clenched fist or a skipped heartbeat. The body isn't only remembering; it's responding, asking for flow, attention, and movement.

Think of water in a stream. It doesn't get stuck unless something blocks its path. The same is true for emotion. We get stuck when we try to think our way through what the body is trying to feel. We ask: *What does this mean?* But the more honest question is: What wants to move? Tightness, restlessness, heat—these aren't problems, they're invitations.

It took years to realize that I didn't need to fix what I felt. I just needed to let it move through me. That's how the F.E.E.L. Method was born: one breath, one sensation, one moment at a time.

THE TOOL

THE F.E.E.L. METHOD

Find • Embody • Express • Let it Move

The F.E.E.L. Method grew out of my own lived experience with grief. Years of learning that emotions aren't problems to solve, but energy asking to move. It's the practice that helped me stay in my body when everything in me wanted to leave it.

It teaches emotional regulation as a relationship rather than control. When we relate to emotion as energy, we stop managing feelings and start collaborating with the body's intelligence.

This is how healing becomes embodied: not all at once, but one sensation at a time, one moment of staying instead of fleeing.

STEP 1: FIND

Bring awareness to what's happening inside.

Notice where the sensation lives in your body: your chest, gut, jaw, or throat.

Ask simple, curious questions:

- What am I noticing here?

- What's its texture: tight, dense, fluttering, still?

- Does it have movement? Does it rise, press, swirl, or pull?

- Does it feel hot and throbbing or cold and still?

When I first tried to 'find' the sensation in my body, it was usually a tightness in my chest, the same one I felt sitting by my mother's hospital bed.

This step is about orientation, not analysis.

Finding the sensation tells your body, I'm here. I'm listening. Awareness itself is the first act of regulation.

STEP 2: EMBODY

Once you locate the sensation, bring it closer instead of pushing it away.

Gently name what you feel and where it lives:

"Fear in my chest."

"Sadness behind my eyes."

"Tightness in my stomach."

Naming gives form to sensation. It creates just enough space between you and the emotion to stay present with it.

This isn't intellectual labeling; it's ownership. You're letting the experience belong to you, instead of treating it as something foreign or dangerous.

STEP 3: EXPRESS

Once you've found and named the sensation, meet it with compassion.

Before you move or act, apply soothing self-talk, the kind you'd offer a child or a friend:

"I see you."

"This is so hard."

"You're safe now."

Let tone and presence do the work. You might place a hand over your heart or wherever the feeling lives.

This isn't about doing something to the feeling; it's about being with it kindly.

When the body feels met, it begins to soften. And in that softening, movement starts to happen on its own.

STEP 4: LET IT MOVE

Every emotion has a natural arc.

When we stop managing it and stop attaching stories or meaning, the body finds its own resolution.

Letting it move might look like:

- a full exhale or spontaneous sigh

- a yawn, a tremor, or tears

- gentle bouncing, swaying, or shaking

- wrapping your arms around yourself

- resting when your body asks for stillness

If the energy feels too strong, titrate, touch in, then step back.

This rhythm between activation and safety is called pendulation. It's how the nervous system learns to trust itself again.

This step isn't about fixing or forcing feelings. It's about allowing energy to move and listening for what completion feels like; the quiet after the wave passes.

Letting go didn't mean forgetting her or the grief. It meant letting the energy move, just as I had to do day after day during those seven years.

Over time, this practice builds capacity to stay present with greater waves of emotion without collapsing or disconnecting.

When I think back to those years with my mom, what I remember most is the constant edge of living grief, holding on while preparing to let go. The way my body carried what words could not.

I didn't have the language then, but what I learned was the experience of felt safety: staying present with what was alive inside me, letting energy move instead of bracing against it.

That's what the F.E.E.L. Method became: a way to stay with myself when everything in me wanted to flee.

It's what I now offer to others, a way back into a relationship with the body, one breath, one sensation, one moment at a time.

You don't have to fix what you feel. You only have to stay with it long enough for it to move.

Every emotion, even grief, is energy looking for a home.

If something stirs as you read this, a tightening, a flutter, a lump in the throat, that's the beginning of the practice.

Don't analyze it. Don't name it—just notice.

And when you can, meet it.

A breath. A hand to your heart. A quiet *I'm here.*

This is where the practice begins in daily life, not in theory, but in the body.

That's the invitation to begin, not by thinking about healing, but by feeling what's already asking to move.

You can start right now. Whatever you notice, however small, let it be enough. Trust that every moment of presence is a step toward healing. Give yourself permission to feel, to move, to be here. Your body already knows the way.

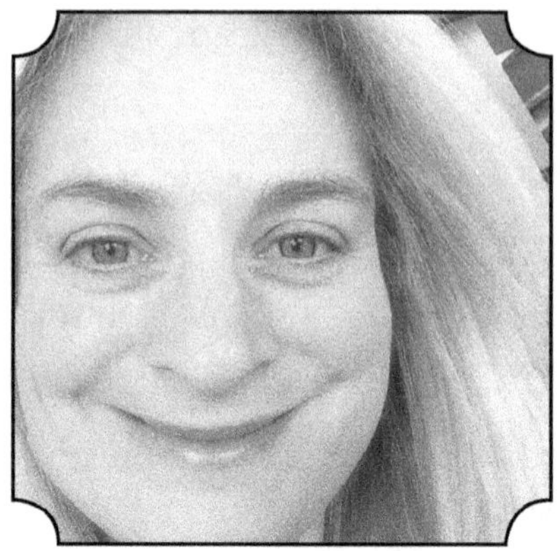

Faith Galliano Desai, Ph.D., is a psychologist, educator, and speaker who invites people to return to themselves, not as a project to fix but as a life to inhabit fully. After more than twenty years in psychology, she has transitioned from direct clinical care to teaching, coaching, and speaking, guiding others to understand the nervous system as a bridge between mind, body, and lived experience.

She works with people who are tired of quick fixes or being defined by trauma, anxiety, or any single part of their story. Faith's approach is about honoring the full sweep of being alive, including grief that lingers, love that surprises, the ache of loss, the search for purpose, and the tension between wanting safety and craving growth. She teaches that emotion is not an enemy to be managed, but a message to be listened to with curiosity rather than control.

What happens in her sessions is not magic. It is the start of an authentic relationship with self. Growth becomes sustainable. People often describe leaving with a clearer sense of what is happening inside, a little more permission to be themselves, less tension in their bodies, and more patience for the hard days. The most common thing people say is that they walk away with practical tools and a fresh sense of possibility, more able to meet themselves with compassion and curiosity.

CONNECT WITH FAITH:

Email: drfaithgallianodesai@icloud.com

LinkedIn: https://www.linkedin.com/in/faithgallianodesai

Trauma imprints itself deep within us,
but it also opens a doorway.

~ Heather Potvin

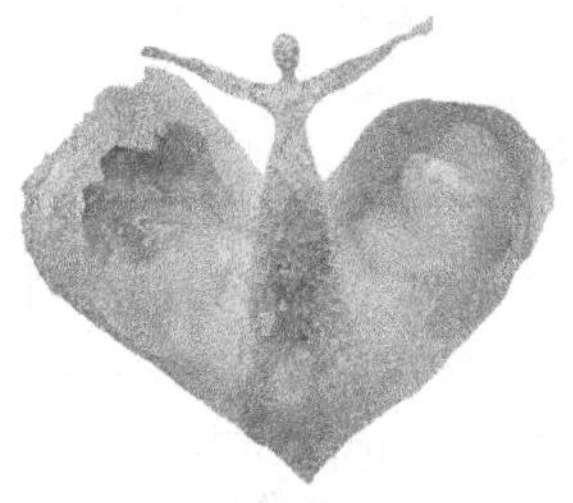

Chapter 19

Journey to Inner Wholeness
Heather's Mind Body Heaven

Heather Potvin

EOLD, Holistic Wellness Advisor

My Story

Traumatic memories can keep us locked in a fight or flight loop that quietly ruins our lives.

The brain can't always tell the difference between a memory and a real event—it accepts everything as truth. When we recall something painful, our brain reacts as if it's happening again and sends signals through the body to respond accordingly. Each stressful thought triggers the body's defense system, creating confusion within our cells and preventing the body from maintaining its natural state of balance and health.

I learned this lesson the hardest way possible.

It began after the passing of my beloved husband, Howie. Each night, as I lay my head on the pillow, I was transported back through the final three years of his life. My mind relived every decision, every conversation with doctors, and every obstacle we faced. *Did I do enough?* In my body, it was as if I was living it all over again—the adrenaline, fear, and fierce determination imprinted deep within my cells.

Catch the cycle in that? Imagine reliving it again and again.

When Howie was diagnosed with Stage 3 cancer of the liver and bile duct, we became warriors together. We researched, questioned, and made changes to everything we could. We eliminated processed foods, explored alternative treatments, and surrounded ourselves with hope. Friends called in favors that led us to City of Hope and one of the best oncology teams available. Our doctor even traveled to New York to learn how to administer the newest immune therapy—a customized cocktail of three drugs designed specifically for Howie's tumors.

Many nights, we lay in bed talking quietly, sometimes in tears, sometimes in laughter. Often, we just held hands. During one of those sacred moments, I asked him gently about his death.

"If you could have your wish," I whispered, "what would your death look like?"

He became quiet. I held his hand and waited. " I know what I don't want," he replied softly.

I took a breath, "Let's start with what don't you want?"

"I don't want to be in a hospital with a bunch of people standing around, waiting for me to die, or crying over me," he remarked, closing his eyes.

"Then what would you want? In an ideal world?"

He paused again as if seeing it in his head. "I would want to be at home, in the living room, in my recliner. Just my girls, no one else. Normal things are going on in the house. The three of you are talking and laughing while I sit in my recliner." Then he inhaled a long, slow breath. "I would just stop breathing," he said.

I looked into his eyes, filled with tears but also with peace.

"If I can make that happen, I will," I promised.

Near the end of COVID, we believed we had beaten the cancer and could finally focus on healing the damage from chemotherapy. But in September 2021, we made our final trip to the hospital. We fought on the way there—both exhausted, both afraid. For twenty-two years, our words to each other had always come from love, and even our anger was rooted in that love.

That Sunday before he passed, I sat on the edge of his hospital bed and held his hand. His voice was soft. "You've always been my rock," he said. "If you're falling apart, what chance do I have?"

This is the man I love with all my heart. I knew then—I needed to be strong, not just for him, but for both of us.

That Sunday, in soft tones, he told me he didn't want to die in the hospital or alone. And I told him, "I won't let that happen."

When I saw the signs that his time was near, I called the hospice team. During COVID, hospitals had strict rules, but I was determined. I muscled my way past security and into his room. If love could've been a weapon, that day I wielded it fiercely. When the hospital mentioned sending a hospital bed, Howie said a firm "No." He wanted his own bed, his own space. Even as his body weakened, his spirit stayed strong.

With hospice guidance, I brought him home—just as he wished.

He was joking with the EMTs as they carried him into the house. One of them laughed, saying, "Your husband is quite the character." My daughter smiled and said, "When he stops making jokes, we know we're in trouble."

Less than twenty hours later, we said goodbye.

One of the last things he said to me was that he wanted to sit in his recliner. That last night, I was exhausted but lay on the couch beside Howie. I held his hand until he fell asleep. His breathing was shallow and labored as he struggled with each inhale. Knowing the next morning was going to be a challenging one, I left him to sleep in our bed. And I prayed his passing would come quickly. *This gentle man doesn't deserve to suffer.*

Early the next morning, I walked into the living room to find him halfway on the floor. In the night, he slipped down in his chair. With considerable effort, I lifted him into a more comfortable sitting position. His eyes were now swollen shut, and his face all but unrecognizable. The swelling now affected his throat, so he could no longer speak. I knew the love of my life didn't have much longer on this Earth. My heart ached for this man.

I called hospice and my daughters. While the nurse was with Howie, I sat in the backyard and prepared our girls for what was to come. Based on her assessment of his condition, the hospice nurse ordered a hospital bed for him.

After the nurse left, my girls and I began discussing how to arrange the room for his last few days. At one point, my oldest daughter turned to look at him. "He's not breathing," she gasped. The man I loved with my whole heart passed exactly the way he wanted.

Traumatic memories can trap us in that loop of fight or flight. What you just read was mine.

For weeks after his passing, I relived that day and the three years before it, repeatedly.

Did I do enough?

Could I have done more?

Did I say enough?

Did I fight hard enough?

And each time, after the storm of questions came the quiet truth: *I did enough. I loved him fully, fiercely, and faithfully.*

That realization marked the first step in my healing.

A close friend stayed with me for the first seventy-two hours and suggested I try a Reiki session to clear my energy. The session brought deep peace during the day, though the nights still tormented me. I was exhausted, caught in a loop of making poor decisions, getting sick again and again. I knew something had to change.

"Why don't you try meditation?" that same friend suggested. I nearly laughed—*been there, done that.* I practiced meditation in the 1970s, but this was different. What I discovered was a way to quiet my mind and stop the relentless images that played every night. This was the first time I realized energy could shift not just my mind, but my body's memory of pain.

A new path opened before me—not only to my own healing, but to helping others find theirs.

Here's what I discovered.

Although it involves a little effort and practice, I promise it has considerably improved my life. Now, I teach this to everyone who needs to change the way their brain communicates with the cells in their body.

The trauma doesn't have to be the loss of a loved one. It can be leaving domestic violence or recovery from substance abuse, or childhood trauma. It can come from the constant stress of your current job.

I recently began working with women recovering from horrific experiences. By providing them with these resources, they can concentrate on advancing in their personal health journey. The first step in each person's recovery process is to shift their mental response from fight or flight to calm and concentration.

A man was referred to me because of his difficulty with flying. The PTSD he carried from the Gulf War made it impossible for him to be in a closed space. He was fine until the airplane doors closed, then the panic would set in. His body shifted into fight or flight mode, and he felt trapped. His coping mechanism was to talk constantly throughout the flight, much to the dismay of the passenger seated next to him.

Once he was in a meditative state, I said, "Try to see an image that evokes a peaceful feeling." As he immersed himself in that image, I watched his facial expressions soften. His breathing slowed. I invited him to focus on what that peace felt like in his body—the physical sensation of calm.

When bringing him back to a waking state, I gave him a cue he could use to recall this image and feeling any time he boarded a plane.

I encouraged him to repeat the steps often, so they'd become part of his body's memory—an anchor to rely on each time he flew.

Grief imprints itself deep within us, but also opens a doorway. Through that doorway, I found the path not only to my own healing—but to helping others find theirs.

My wish for you is that you feel peace, love, and calm deep within your cells, that you'll learn to change the conversation between your mind and your body.

The Tool

Your First Steps to Wholeness

First, find a quiet time. For many of my clients, the evening is the best quiet time. For some of my clients, it's the morning, before the tiny humans wake up.

Find a quiet place and make yourself comfortable.

Sitting in a secure chair with head support is important.

Lying on the floor, on a couch, or on your bed is often best.

Once you're settled, close your eyes and let your attention rest on the next few steps.

If it helps, you can follow along with the guided audio linked in this chapter.

Remember, there's no wrong way to do this.

Each time you practice, you build a bridge between your mind and your body.

Every session brings more ease and a deeper connection.

Take **two quick breaths in** through your mouth.
Then **one long, slow breath out.**

This simple rhythm reconnects the brain with the body's electrical signals—a technique known as the **Vagus Nerve Reset** or **Vagus Nerve Stimulator.**

Now take a **deep breath in** through your nose, filling your lungs completely.
Hold for a count of three.
Then **release the air through your mouth,** emptying your lungs fully, and hold for another count of three before repeating.
As you breathe, focus on how the air feels—cool as it enters your nostrils, moving down the back of your throat, expanding your lungs. Feel the warmth as it leaves your body.

Repeat the deep, slow breathing three to five more times, keeping your focus on your breath. Each inhale fills you with calm and peace. Each exhale releases stress and tension.

If a negative thought enters your mind, imagine wrapping it gently in a cocoon—or placing it in a container that feels right for you. Then, release it with your next exhale.

For me, that container is a **balloon,** floating away with the wind.
For you, it might be **bubbles,** drifting, and dissolving.

Shift your focus to your heart rate as you slow your breathing down. Imagine your heartbeat and the blood flowing freely through your body. This visualization may take practice, but you can do it.

Next, shift your focus to your **muscles.**
Start with your toes.
Notice how they feel—warm, cool, tight, or relaxed.
Picture your toes in a state of comfort and ease.

Slowly move your attention upward to your feet, ankles, calves, and thighs.
Then your hips, your abdomen, your chest.
Continue to your shoulders, arms, and hands.
Up your neck, your jaw, your face, all the way to the crown of your head.

With each breath, soften each muscle.
Let your body release what it no longer needs to hold.
Take your time—there's no rush, no time limit.

When you reach the top of your head, your body should feel **peaceful and still.**
Your mind should feel **clear and open.**

It's time to work with your brain and gently shift the conversation it has with your body.

Picture a moment in your life when you felt complete joy and happiness. This could be any moment—big or small. See it clearly in your mind's eye. Who is there? What are you doing? Allow yourself to fully feel each emotion. Let that feeling spread through your entire body. Hold this image in your mind. This will become your signal, a touchstone you can call upon whenever you wish to guide your body into a state of peace.

Each time you experience a negative thought or emotion, call upon this image to restore your body to a state of calm and peace. Again, it may take practice, but I know you can do it

Now, let's create a sense of protection for this peaceful state.

Think about a color, any color that evokes the same emotion. This color is **yours.** The color for me is a gentle violet. This color always makes me feel at ease and content. Select yours. How does it appear? Is it sturdy? Does this color's depth vary in any way? Does it shimmer or sparkle? What shape does it have? See it as you would like it to be.

Now visualize the color radiating up through the top of your head, drifting downward around your entire head. See it float down over your shoulders, heart space, and arms. Moving fluidly down over your torso, your legs, and all the way to your feet.

See it expanding out around your entire body. Nothing negative can penetrate this color field. You can see through it, extend your peaceful energy beyond it. This is your safe space.

Each time you experience a negative thought or emotion, call upon this image to restore your body to a state of calm and peace. Again, it may take practice, but I know you can do it.

You may need a physical trigger, such as touching your thumb and forefinger. You may need to do the double breath (Vegas Nerve Reset). Pick one that works for you.

Once you've mastered this first step in establishing a healthy connection between your brain and body, you may want to explore how to use this to work on specific areas of your body for improved health. This technique is an excellent addition to other forms of healing, such as a balanced diet, regular exercise, energy work, and counseling.

HERE ARE THE STEPS:

1. Find a quiet space and a comfortable, safe position.

2. Take two quick breaths in and one long, slow breath out to do the Vegas Nerve Reset and open communication to the body.

3. A series of deep breaths as described above, three to five times.

4. Continue with the deep breathing as you focus on softening each part of your body. Remember to take each breath slowly to promote a state of peace.

5. Visualize a time in your life that brings you joy and peace. Imprint that feeling into your cells.

6. Choose a color as a reminder of the feelings you just imprinted into your body. This is your cue.

7. See and feel that color covers your entire body, protecting you and keeping you safe.

8. Slowly return to your body, move your toes and fingers. Move your feet and arms. Stretch. Move your shoulders and your head.

I encourage you to practice this meditation each morning when you wake up and each night before you go to sleep. Eventually, the visualization will become a part of you. You can then add words of encouragement and gratitude. I find repeating them during the day very helpful, and you may find the same.

You are an amazing, beautiful Soul.

The strength inside you is more than you feel right now.

You didn't give up.

You are safe, seen, and loved.

You are worthy.

You are on your own personal journey of healing, and you are where you are supposed to be.

Universe, show me how good it can get.

I say three to five of these every day during my meditation.

If you would like to go deeper, explore this on a personal level, schedule a free consultation with me. Heather@nlitepassage.net

Click on this link to download an audio version of this first step: https://enlightenedpassage.net/contact

Remember, you're an amazing, beautiful soul. You're on your own personal journey of healing, and you're exactly where you are supposed to be.

Trauma imprints itself deep within us, but it also opens a doorway. Through that doorway, I found the path not only to my own healing.

My wish for you is to find your own open doorway and the journey to wholeness.

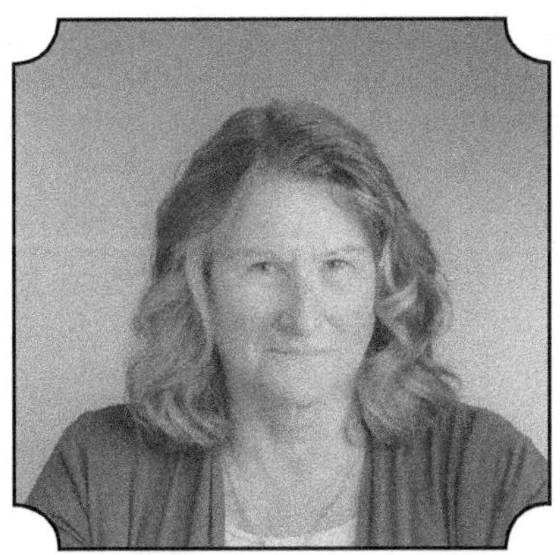

With the death of her cherished husband, Howie, **Heather Potvin** experienced a re-awakening. Her journey toward alternative health began in 1985 when her son was diagnosed with ADHD. This necessitated searching for alternative treatments outside conventional medicine. She has assisted numerous souls in leaving this life over the last 40 years. It wasn't until her husband passed in 2021 that she became certified as an End of Life Doula. Next came certification in energy and sound treatment, and how energy affects the body. After that, she added hypnotherapy and Neuro-Linguistic Programming (NLP) to her list of certificates. Finally, she added Reiki Master to her list of abilities. She developed her meditation treatment technique as a result of all of this instruction, mentoring, and experience.

She believes the road to health is unique for each client. Every motivation is different. They are all connected by one thing. They want to get better. If they can change what they feed their thoughts, they can change how they feed their bodies. This strengthens the body's natural ability to mend itself. Heather's interest is assisting people in achieving balance in their own bodies.

If you find yourself trapped in your own loop—reliving moments of loss, pain, or regret—please know you're not broken. Your body is simply trying to protect you from something your mind still believes is happening. With compassion, awareness, and gentle practices like Reiki, breathwork, or meditation, you can teach your body that it's safe again. Healing doesn't erase the past; it releases its hold on the present.

There is life—and love—waiting beyond the loop.

CONNECT WITH HEATHER:

Website http://www.enlightenedpassage.net/

Email: Heather@nlitepassage.net

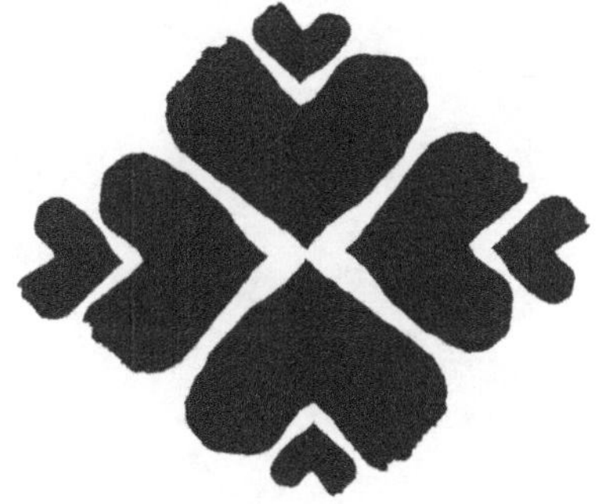

OTHER POSSIBILITIES FOR HEALING

The room went quiet in the way sacred spaces do—everyone smiling that yep, the Universe is winking. That was the evening I stopped pretending these were 'only' pretty cards. They were mirrors and messengers.

~ DeeAnna Merz Nagel

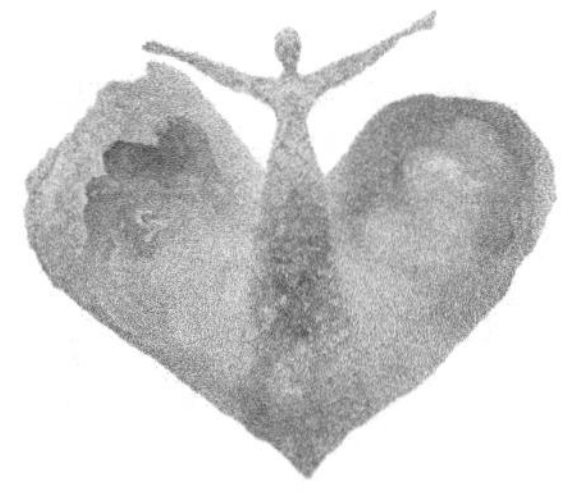

CHAPTER 20

ESSENTIAL SOUL CARE®

DAILY SACRED RITUALS TO SUPPORT YOUR HEALING JOURNEY

DeeAnna Merz Nagel

D.TH, LMHC

**"Stars ink your fingers
with a lexicon of flame
blazing rare knowledge."**
~Aberjhani, The River of Winged Dreams

MY STORY

My eyes watered, the back of my neck tingled, and I really didn't know if I was laughing or crying. I was a bit scared and totally amazed at the same time.

Seriously? You can't make this shit up! This is unbelievably on-point. What's happening here?

Several years ago, by fluke—or more likely, by divine orchestration—the Universe surrounded me with a group of wonderful women. Each month, we gathered for our moon circle, each woman bringing her favorite oracle deck to share. Up to that point, I hadn't paid much attention to the explosion of decks on the market. I was more familiar with Tarot and even took a course on it. But those archetypes and wands and swords didn't speak to me, not like this.

These oracle decks were something else entirely. Each one carried a different energy, a different language of symbols, colors, and archetypes. Every meeting, we spread the cards across the table and gasped at how accurate and aligned the messages were. Sometimes we pulled from more than one deck, layering meanings. Other times, one card was enough to spark deep reflection and laughter. The synchronicities were too strong to ignore. We witnessed something much bigger than coincidence, a kind of sacred choreography arranging itself right in our living room. Over time, I realized that we weren't just reading cards; we were reading energy, consciousness, ourselves.

One night, as candles breathed their soft halos against the wall, I pulled a card about thresholds just hours after signing a new office lease. The image—a door with light spilling under it—felt so literal it almost made me roll my eyes. Minutes later, another woman pulled a card with the same primary symbol from a completely different deck. The room went quiet in the way sacred spaces do—everyone smiling that yep, the Universe is winking. That was the evening I stopped pretending these were "only" pretty cards. They were mirrors and messengers.

I didn't understand the mechanism, but I was hooked. I wanted to know more. So when I learned about a three-day conference hosted by one of my favorite oracle deck creators, I signed up. I thought I'd learn about spreads and symbols. Instead, I found myself on the threshold of a spiritual awakening.

Why are we walking in a circle, chanting? What's all this about mediumship? Am I in the right place?

Yes, I was. And I was about to learn just how much more there was to all of this. For three days, I was immersed in an atmosphere alive with talk of vibration, frequency, ascension, clair senses, and manifestation. The skeptic in me raised an eyebrow, but another part—the intuitive part I'd been suppressing—felt completely at home. Something inside whispered: *Pay attention. This is real.*

The workshop didn't just introduce new concepts—it expanded the boundaries of what I thought was possible. I realized these tools weren't about predicting the future; they were ways of conversing with Spirit.

I already worked with essential oils in my daily life, both for wellness and emotional support. The women in my moon circle brought their cards; I brought my oils. So when I learned about pairing scent with intention in the workshop, it felt like coming home. The facilitator explained, "People often fail to become what they desire because they can't feel that future yet. Sensory experience can anchor us to the past or lead us toward the future." That made total sense to me.

After that, I experimented. I chose a specific oil or blend for each intention I set—financial abundance, courage, peace. Every time I revisited that same intention, I used the same oil. Over time, the scent itself became a bridge between thought and embodiment. Smelling that oil reminded me of what I called in. It became a kind of olfactory affirmation—proof that my senses could work in service of my spirit.

I kept small bottles in my bag the way some people carry talismans. Clary sage before difficult conversations, a bright citrus when I wanted to write with verve, a grounded resin to help me close sessions without carrying everyone's pain home. It wasn't about magic thinking; it was about state training. The scent reminded my nervous system which door to open.

That workshop confirmed my intuitive sense of essential oils, expanded my understanding of oracle decks, and left me with three takeaways that have become part of my philosophy of living:

1. Co-create with Spirit.

2. Don't look for a fortune-teller—create your own future.

3. Anchor your intentions through your senses.

Co-creating with Spirit meant I could stop muscling my way through every transformation and start listening for collaboration. Creating my own future placed me in the posture of an author rather than a passive audience member. And anchoring through my senses became the stealth superpower—building new neural grooves with tangible cues I could repeat.

That weekend was a hinge moment in my life. I was already established as a psychotherapist, coach, and educator. But something deeper called. I came out of what I jokingly called my "pixie closet," acknowledging that my intuitive side was not separate from my professional life—it was essential to it.

To be sure, the path was already widening prior to the workshop. I had enrolled in Reiki training, took chakra classes, revisited Tarot, and kept exploring, all while maintaining a busy private practice and supervising other therapists. Then, a friend introduced me to essential oils, and that became a whole new chapter. For a few years, I focused on teaching others the benefits of essential oils. I was going through a huge personal transition—separating from my husband, moving back to my home state, reconfiguring my entire career. I even opened a brick-and-mortar aromatherapy boutique for a time, a tiny temple of scent and conversation where people came for oils and left having set intentions. It's where those moon circles began.

And that was the beginning of what became *Essential Soul Care®*: the book, the oracle deck, and the course. Once I committed to writing, everything began to unfold in ways I couldn't have planned. I invited my colleague Madison to collaborate. We're alike in our foundations but bring different gifts to the table. Together, we wrote *The Essential Soul Care® Playbook: Designing an Expansive Life.*

We called it a playbook intentionally. I wanted people to exhale when they opened it—a place to try on practices without evaluation, to move ink around on paper until the soul's voice got louder than the inner critic. The Playbook explores the seven elements of soul expansion and their alignment with the seven chakras:

- Transcendence—Crown

- Intuition—Third Eye

- Mindset—Throat

- Community—Heart

- Nourishment—Solar Plexus

- Creativity—Sacral

- Sanctuary—Root

Each element is paired with tools—essential oils, crystals, affirmations, journal prompts, and reflective exercises. The goal is to make the invisible visible—to bridge energy and emotion with tangible daily practice.

We wrote at my kitchen table, with mugs of tea and sticky notes multiplying like butterflies. We asked questions like, "What does the heart want someone to practice when the world feels unkind?" and "How can the root feel like a sanctuary when life is anything but?" We drafted exercises people could do in five minutes or in an afternoon, because healing needs to fit inside ordinary days.

But as soon as we finished, I knew there was more to be done.

*I wonder how Madison's gonna react when I spring **this** on her?*

I told her, "*The Playbook* needs a companion oracle deck." She didn't hesitate. Within days, we channeled forty-nine messages and images that flowed so effortlessly we couldn't even tell who wrote what. We found an artist who captured our vision beautifully—simple, monochromatic imagery that expressed our concept of sacred symbolism.

I still remember the moment the number 49 clicked—seven by seven, a perfect square of wholeness. The deck wanted to be a map and a mirror. Each card became a small doorway: an archetypal image, a distilled message, and an invitation to act. When we held the first printed proofs, I felt the same neck-tingle I had in that very first moon circle. The oracle wasn't just art; it was a living conversation.

Still, something whispered: *Not done yet.*

I realized that these tools weren't just for personal growth; they could serve as therapeutic instruments. That's when The Essential Soul Care® Practitioner Course was born—a 30-hour training in oracle card mastery through symbol and metaphor. It teaches therapists, coaches, and healers how to use these practices in their sessions to help clients engage their own inner wisdom and self-healing.

When I look back now, I see how it all fits together—the psychotherapist, the coach, the aromatherapist, the intuitive, the writer. Every chapter of my life has led here. Essential Soul Care® is not a single thing. It's a living lexicon—a way of listening to the soul's language through image, scent, intuition, and reflection.

I came full circle, right back to that first moon circle—only now, I understood that the cards, the oils, the rituals were never the point. They were portals.

THE TOOL

Essential Soul Care® is one tool among many—a living, breathing practice composed of sensory, creative, and spiritual experiences that help you reconnect with yourself. There's no one-size-fits-all formula. Instead, it's a collection of invitations and ways to experiment with your own energy, creativity, and awareness.

Labyrinth (the spiral path back to Self). When life feels chaotic, try tracing a labyrinth. Use your finger on paper or walk a life-sized one if you have access. Follow its winding path inward and pause at the center. Breathe. Listen. Notice what arises. Then, as you move outward, imagine releasing what no longer serves you. The labyrinth teaches us that healing isn't linear—it's spiraled, cyclical, alive.

Deepen it: before you begin, name your intention in a single sentence. At the center, place one hand on your heart and ask, What is the next kind step? On the way out, exhale audibly with each turn to "unhook" the residue. If walking a physical labyrinth, let your pace change naturally—fast around one curve, slow on another. Your nervous system will often choose what it needs.

Scent (state training for the nervous system). If your energy feels heavy, invite scent into your practice. Choose an essential oil that reflects your desired state—lavender for peace, peppermint for clarity, geranium for love. As you inhale, affirm your intention. The scent becomes a bridge between what you imagine and what you embody. Over time, your body will remember that feeling before your mind does.

Deepen it: pair one intention with one scent for at least 21 days. Keep the bottle near the place you practice (desk, altar, nightstand). Whisper the same short phrase each time—"I speak clearly," "I am safe in my body," "I choose gentleness." Consider a patch test and appropriate dilution; your ritual should feel supportive, not overwhelming.

Oracle (dialogue, not prediction). When you want guidance, pull a daily oracle card. Don't ask for predictions. Instead, ask, "What do I need to know today?" Let the imagery and message sit with you. Write about it if you wish. Sometimes the insight comes immediately; other times, it reveals itself later through synchronicity.

Deepen it: try a three-card "Now / Next / Nourish" spread. "Now" names the energy you're in. "Next" points toward a micro-action. "Nourish" suggests how to care for yourself while you act. In sessions, position the card between you and a client to externalize stuck material; it becomes the safe third thing you can both reference without defensiveness.

Writing (ink as portal). Contemplative writing isn't about journaling every detail of your day—it's about listening to your inner wisdom without editing. Try prompts like 'What wants to be known today?' or 'What am I resisting that's trying to love me?' Pair that with a gratitude journal to keep your heart tuned to expansion, and a synchronicity journal to record those winks from the Universe—the songs, numbers, or chance meetings that affirm you're on the right path.

Deepen it: set a seven-minute timer and write without lifting your pen. When the critic interrupts, write, "and what I really mean is. . ." and keep going. End each entry with one sentence that begins, "I'm willing to. . ." It gently moves reflection toward embodied choice.

Haiku (the discipline of tenderness). When emotions feel tangled, try writing a haiku. Its 5-7-5 structure invites simplicity and precision. Limitations can be liberating. A few words can hold a lifetime of feeling.

Wilted flower bends—
Water, light, and time restore.
Blossoming again.

Deepen it: write three haiku on the same feeling: one naming the ache, one naming the resource, one naming the next right step. Pin your favorite where you'll see it—on the kettle, the mirror, the laptop lid—so your day keeps reminding you.

Play (joy as medicine). Don't forget the healing power of play. Deep work and play are partners, not opposites. Coloring, puzzles, collage, dancing, or doodling—all these activities balance the right and left brain and reawaken joy. Healing doesn't always happen in silence; sometimes it happens through laughter and motion.

Deepen it: keep a "joy kit" nearby: crayons, washi tape, a glue stick, a tiny stack of magazine cut-outs, a deck of your favorite cards. When your mind spirals, spend five minutes making a nonsensical collage. The goal is delight, not perfection.

***

These small, accessible practices—the labyrinth, the scent, the oracle, the writing, the poetry, and the play—are all facets of Essential Soul Care®. Use them like keys to unlock your own insight. Mix and match. Follow what expands you. What soothes one day may not the next, and that's okay. The work is to keep listening.

Over time, these practices become spiritual muscle memory. You start to recognize when you're contracting and when you're expanding. You begin to notice that peace has a rhythm, and joy has a frequency. These tools train you not to escape your life, but to inhabit it more fully.

Essential Soul Care® reminds us that self-care isn't a luxury; it's an act of communication with your higher self. It's how you say, "I'm here. I'm listening." Each ritual—each breath, scent, card, or word—is a love letter to your own becoming. So begin where you are. Maybe today, it's three mindful breaths and a drop of lavender on your wrist. Maybe tomorrow, it's a journal entry or a walk in the moonlight. Whatever you choose, let it be playful. Let it be yours.

What simple, expansive tool could you play with today to hear what it unlocks for you?

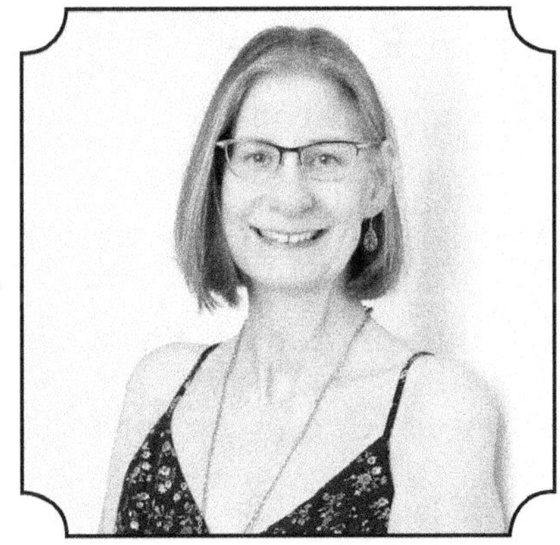

Dr. DeeAnna Merz Nagel is a seasoned psychotherapist, clinical supervisor, coach, and aromatherapist. Her work is deeply influenced by an intuitive perspective, with teaching being the core aspect of her current endeavors. With over 30 years of experience in direct service to individuals, families, and groups, she is now solely and soulfully dedicated to facilitating learning in the healing arts and sharing insights from her own direct experiences. She guides practitioners on clinical, psycho-spiritual, and intuitive learning journeys!

DeeAnna aspires to guide individuals as they learn to guide others, whether it be as therapists, coaches, energy healers, or intuitive practitioners. She is eager to help practitioners incorporate alternative approaches into their practice. She aims to serve as a gatekeeper to the counseling profession by providing skilled, synergistic clinical supervision and training and helping practitioners integrate metaphysical, psycho-spiritual, and subtle energy methods into their client work. She creates professional development experiences that seamlessly align with personal growth.

DeeAnna co-created Essential Soul Care®, a psycho-spiritual model featuring a course, a book, and an oracle deck with Dr. Madison Leigh Akridge. She has authored several other books, book chapters, and articles. Her work has garnered recognition in national publications such as the New York Times, USA Today, and Women's Health.

CONNECT WITH DEEANNA:

Website: https://deeannamerznagel.com

Information about Essential Soul Care®:
https://deeannamerznagel.com/essential-soul-care/

Instagram: https://www.instagram.com/deeannanagel

YouTube: https://www.youtube.com/@DeeAnnaNagel

X: https://x.com/DeeAnnaNagel

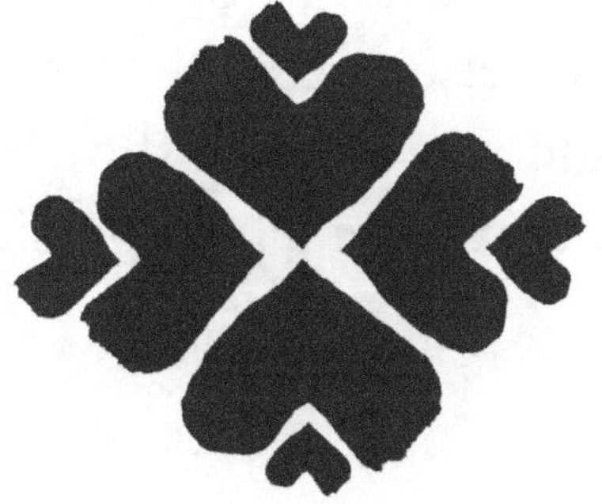

You're allowed to change, become something
new, and return to something old.
You can imagine new ways of showing up in the
world that once felt impossible.

~ April Hannah

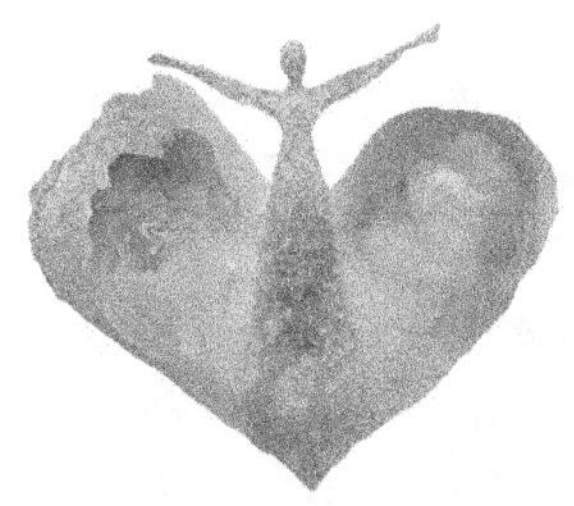

Chapter 21

The I AM Affirmation Method
A Creative Path to Confidence and Fearless Living

April Hannah

MS.ED., LMHCD, RMT

My Story

I AM not good enough.
I AM never going to be a Reiki Master Teacher.
I AM not a filmmaker.
I AM not a podcast host.
I AM never going to do mental health therapy again.
I AM not an artist.
I AM not a sound healer.
I AM not a retreat facilitator.
I AM not an author.

Or so I thought.

Words cast spells, and in the words of Henry Ford, "Whether you think you can or you think you can't, you're right."

The day I realized the words I thought and spoke could affect my very cells, and the experiences I drew into my life, was over lunch in a

Manhattan restaurant with a close friend 28 years ago. We were both in our late twenties, already on our spiritual paths. I just finished my Level 1 Reiki training, and together we had a handful of psychic and tarot readings and shared the same spiritual advisor.

I can still picture that day clearly. It was a chilly fall Friday in October. I took my own mental health day from my private practice and planned a girls' day out with one of my best friends, Mary. She lived closer to the city, so we always made an adventure out of our visits. We'd take the Metro-North train from Beacon, New York, to Grand Central Terminal, find a fancy restaurant where we could be foodies, grab a delicious, overpriced cocktail that we'd never make for ourselves, and pretend we were one of the girls in the sitcom *Sex and the City*. As soon as we arrived, we'd dash off the train, climb the subway stairs two at a time, and step into the dopamine rush of Manhattan.

We had a ritual: Wander until a restaurant "found" us. That day, we sat down at a chic, bougie restaurant downtown. Our get-togethers were one of those girlfriend lunches where the waiter came by three times before we even looked at the menu. Each time, we looked up at the waiter, laughed, apologized, and said in unison:

"We're sorry, we haven't even looked at the menu yet." Then we turned and looked at one another and shouted, "Jinx, you owe me a Coke!" And laughed some more.

After we placed our order, Mary leaned in closer to me so the couple next to us couldn't eavesdrop, her voice lowered with excitement and whispered,

"I just read *The Hidden Messages in Water* by Dr. Masaru Emoto. He taped words onto petri dishes of water. Positive ones like *love* and *gratitude,* and negative ones like *hate.* When he froze them, the water exposed to positive words formed beautiful crystalline shapes. The negative words? Just blobs." Then her eyes widened, and she sat back to take in my reaction.

My eyes widened as well, and my jaw dropped. I spoke my thoughts out loud,

"Oh no! Could all the negative self-talk I've been repeating in my head for years actually be affecting my body? After all, the human body is mostly made up of water."

This ignited a conversation that lasted the entire day. When I got home, I immediately sat down at my computer, typed "Messages in Water photos" into Google, and hit enter. My heart pounded as the images appeared. The word *love* created a perfect, snowflake-like crystal. But *I hate you* looked like an ugly blob, just like Mary said. From that moment on, I spoke and thought with intention. I changed my internal thoughts from *I'm not good enough* to *I can do anything I put my mind to,* and *if other people have done it, then I can do it too.*

My curiosity deepened after I read Dr. Emoto's book, leading me to read 40 books written by Wayne Dyer and listen to hours of his YouTube lectures. If you don't know the work of Wayne Dyer, you should. Wayne was a self-help author and motivational speaker, often called the "Father of Motivation," known for his books on self-development and spiritual growth. He spoke passionately about the *I AM* vibration, calling those two words the most powerful in the human language. He referenced scripture in the book of Exodus in the Old Testament of *I AM* being the words that God spoke when Moses asked for God's name, and countless examples of people transforming their lives, including his own, by simply affirming what came after *I AM.*

Throughout history, *I AM* has appeared in spiritual and metaphysical texts as a declaration of identity, existence, and divine connection. These words influence reality through intention. They affirm our higher self, the infinite, creative intelligence within.

While listening to an *I AM* inspired musical track Wayne created, called the "I Am wishes Fulfilled Meditation", I remembered a moment four years earlier when my Reiki master teacher said,

"April, I know you'll be a great Reiki master teacher someday."

I laughed and replied, "I have no desire to become a Reiki master teacher."

After listening to that meditation, I broke that spell and said to myself, "*I AM* ready to become a Reiki master teacher," and within a month, I completed my training and began teaching. Since then, I've trained over 200 Reiki students.

However, I wasn't always consistent with my *I AM* practice. When I wasn't practicing it, heavy self-doubt crept in, especially when I was challenged to try something new or, more recently, when asked to write about my mother's tragic death in my first collaborative book, *The Grief Experience*. The fear of fully stepping into the lifelong goal I had of becoming an author was paralyzing, but I pushed through, cast another spell, and said, "*I AM* an author."

Let's pause for a second and rewind to 2019, when my mother died. Her death shattered me into pieces like a mirror falling off a wall and crashing to the floor. Her death took away my will to continue as a mental health therapist. I decided to retire and shift fully into sound healing, a field that felt both nurturing and expansive, and allowed me to share healing energy without words with my community. My wellness studio was already home to Reiki, meditation classes, women's circles, and spiritual book clubs. But my grief drained my energy. I no longer had the stamina to hold space for others the way I once did.

So, I dove into sound healing during the pandemic. I took every sound healing training available and invested thousands of dollars in instruments. But as my collection of instruments grew, I outgrew my small, 250 sq. ft office and moved into a 1,500-square-foot studio.

Then the fearful thought crept in:

I AM not going to be able to afford this or do this alone.

That thought cast another spell and made me forget my own strength, spiraling me into panic. I began to react out of fear instead of aligned intention. I rushed and invited six other practitioners to teach classes at my studio, but the energy never quite aligned. So, I reinvented the space once more, turned my wellness studio into a sound-healing studio, and pared down to work with two practitioners instead of six. For the next year, I felt like I was on a turbulent roller coaster. The ride was fast, full of unexpected twists and turns. I felt I was losing control. The tracks gave way, the roller coaster derailed, and everything crashed to a halt. The two practitioners jumped off and left abruptly without warning. The ride was over, and I was left alone, standing in the wreckage to pick up all the pieces, questioning everything all over again.

Now what do I do?

Do I really enjoy being just a sound healer? Do I want to continue running a sound healing studio alone?

The answer to these questions came back with a loud, **NO.** The power of the *I AM* rose within me again.

Why did I let go of everything I loved? I am also a therapist, filmmaker, artist, Reiki master teacher, author, and podcast host. How could I limit myself to just one title?

That's when I heard a voice outside of me, "You are still all of these things."

I knew that voice. It guided me two months before my mother died, and helped me save my business from closing during COVID. That voice has never steered me wrong. When that voice speaks, I listen.

With the help of that inner voice and my husband and close friends, I faced the uncomfortable truth: I would have to redefine myself **again.** What looked like failure was actually an invitation to reconnect with my soul and remember who I really was. In the middle of that busy summer after the roller coaster crashed, I successfully ran my studio alone for another year, sold out classes, and made the unthinkable decision to close my sound-healing studio.

I AM done running a wellness studio.

Within a month, I held a closing ceremony and hired a marketing team to help me clarify my vision to integrate all of my *I AMs* under one umbrella. During one of those strategy calls, I heard the familiar voice say:

"You will teach people about the power of *I AM.*"

I shared what I heard with the team, and in a few days, we gathered again on a Zoom call, and they presented me with an *I AM* logo that immediately made my heart swell with love. I knew I was coming home to myself, to wholeness, and knew I had the strength to run my business alone. Just me and my community.

Now, I can say with confidence and fearless conviction:

I AM good enough.
I AM—and always will be— a mental health therapist at the core.
I AM a Reiki Master Teacher.
I AM a filmmaker.
I AM a podcast host.
I AM an artist.
I AM a sound healer.
I AM a retreat facilitator.
I AM an author.
I AM a teacher.
I AM a guide who helps others find their own I AM.

What I have learned along my *I AM* journey is that it's never static; it's always in motion. You're allowed to change, become something new, and return to something old. You can imagine new ways of showing up in the world that once felt impossible.

In my journal, one of my future affirmations reads:

I AM a musician who makes music and has an album.

That dream still feels distant, but then again, I once thought I'd never be any of the things I am today. If I can become all of this, then you can too simply by speaking and writing your truth into existence.

THE TOOL

Say it. Believe it. Become it.

The words you repeat every day become the stories you live. When I began experimenting with the words *I AM,* I quickly learned that they weren't just affirmations; they were energetic declarations. *I AM* is not a wish or a hope; it's a statement of being. It's the language your subconscious and your energy field understand.

Every time you say *I AM,* you instruct your body, emotions, and the universe to align with that frequency. Whether you say I *AM t*ired or *I AM* powerful, your cells and your surroundings begin to respond. This is why so many spiritual teachers, from ancient mystics to modern psychologists, remind us to speak life into our existence.

Over the years, I refined this understanding into a 3-step process I developed called **The *I AM* Affirmation Method.**

STEP ONE: AWARENESS

The first step is becoming aware of the inner dialogue that runs through your mind all day long. We think about 60,000 to 70,000 thoughts a day, and most of them are repetitive, negative, and rooted in fear, comparison, or old stories that no longer serve us.

When you catch yourself thinking, *I'm not good enough* or *I'm an anxious person,* pause and notice it. Awareness alone begins to shift energy. You cannot change a thought you're not aware of.

When I teach this method to my online *I AM* Circle community, I invite people to carry a notebook or use the notes app on their phone for one day. Each time they notice a limiting thought, they simply write it down. By the end of the day, most are surprised to see how often their *I AM* statements are actually *I AM* not statements.

Once you've noticed your limiting language, ask yourself these three questions:

- What do I want to believe about myself instead?

- How do I want to feel when I wake up in the morning?

- Who am I choosing to become?

Your *I AM* statement should feel slightly beyond your current reality—something that stretches you, just like the one in my journal today: *I am a musician who makes music and has an album.* That is still believable because I am a sound healer, own a variety of instruments, and can put notes together that sound like songs. My mind and body won't reject this thought because I'm already halfway there.

STEP TWO: INTEGRATION THROUGH JOURNALING

Writing your *I AM* statements anchors them into the physical world. The act of putting pen to paper moves the energy out of your head and into visible form. Each time you write, you give your subconscious new evidence to work with. That's why I created the *Awakening Your I AM Affirmation Journey* that you can buy on Amazon. It gives people a simple, consistent way to practice this daily.

When you write your affirmations, don't worry if you don't believe them yet. Fake it until you make it, and let your *I AM* evolve into your new truth. Some days it might be *"I AM* healing." Other days, it might be *"I AM* complete," or *"I AM* resting." Every affirmation carries its own vibration, and each one is sacred.

STEP THREE: REFLECTION AND RENEWAL

At the end of each month, reflection closes the energetic loop. It allows you to witness how much you've grown and to celebrate the ways your affirmation has begun to take a life of its own in your life.

This is why the End-of-Month Reflection Exercise is so important. It transforms your practice from a list of affirmations into a personal evolution map. You begin to see the invisible become visible in the small shifts in thought, the quiet moments of courage, the fears you begin to conquer, and the way your energy begins to change the energy around you.

THE CREATIVE EXPANSION: THE *I AM* WHEEL

Because creativity and spirituality are so deeply connected, I developed the *I AM* Wheel as a bonus step to this method. The wheel is a visual and artistic extension of this work to get your creative juices flowing. The *I AM* Wheel invites you to color, draw, paint, or collage your affirmations into a full-circle representation of your becoming. It engages your right brain—your intuitive, imaginative side—and helps your left brain root the *I AM* statements in a deeper level. You can download your free copy of the *I AM* Wheel on my website.

The *I AM* affirmations are reminders of your inner strength. When you practice the *I AM* Affirmation Method, you train your nervous system to stay grounded in self-worth even when fear, grief, or doubt arise, or you find yourself on a crazy roller coaster ride.

You will notice subtle yet profound changes with this method:
- You speak more kindly to yourself and recover from setbacks quickly.

- You attract experiences that reflect your worth.

- You start to dream bigger, love deeper, and take bolder action.

That is the power of *I AM*.

BEGIN YOUR 30-DAY PRACTICE.

Below are the daily and monthly prompts to help you start your *I AM* journey. I challenge you to commit to this practice for 30 days. At the end of the month, use the reflection exercise to notice how you feel, what changed, and how your energy has shifted. Then consider purchasing the physical journal so you can carry this practice throughout the year and access the yearly goals and end-of-year reflection prompts. I have created the *Awaken Your I AM Affirmation Journey,* available on Amazon, if you'd like to turn this into a full-year practice. But you don't have to wait; you can begin right now.

TODAY'S *I AM*

Affirmation: ____
(Write your chosen statement for the day. One that uplifts, grounds, or inspires you.)

Today I Choose To: ____
(What action, mindset, or energy will support your affirmation?)

Evidence of My Confidence Today: ____________________________
(Notice even the smallest ways you showed up with courage or authenticity.)

A Fear I Released or Faced Today: _______________________________
(What belief or story lost its power today?)

Reflections or Insights: _______________________________
(How did your *I AM* shape your experience today?)

END-OF-MONTH REFLECTION EXERCISE

This Month's I AM Was: _______________________________

How I Embodied This Affirmation: _______________________________
(Describe moments when you lived as your I AM self.)

What I Learned About Myself: _______________________________

Fears or Doubts I Released: _______________________________

Ways My Confidence Grew: _______________________________

Favorite Moment or Breakthrough This Month: _______________________________

Next Month, *I AM:* _______________________________

TAKING YOUR I AM INTO THE WORLD

To go even deeper, I've created a fun way to help you spread and inspire the I AM out into the world with the *I AM* Clothing Line so you can literally wear your affirmation, allowing it to vibrate through your body and remind your cells who you are.

When you speak it, write it, feel it, and wear it, your I *AM* becomes your frequency. And when your frequency changes, your entire life begins to shift.

So today, ask yourself one simple question:

Who am I choosing to become? And then answer it with the power, love, and confidence of your truest self: *I AM.*

You don't need to walk this journey alone. I am ready to help you remember who you are. Meet me on my website or social media so we can do this together. I will leave you with my favorite Wayne Dyer quote, "You are always one choice away from a different life." Choose your I *AM a*ffirmation and meet me online!

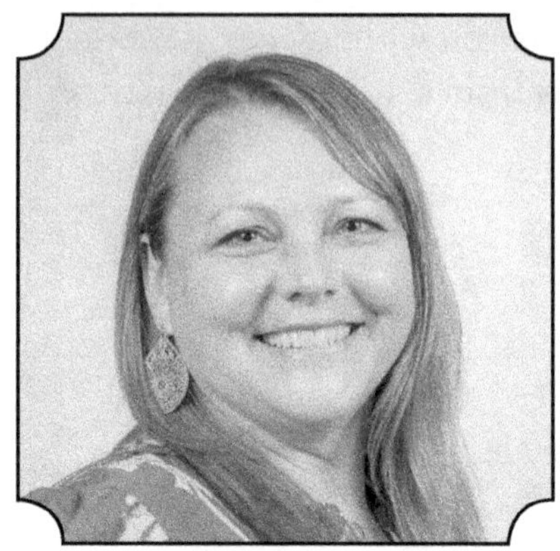

I AM **April Anne Hannah,** a mental health therapist, Reiki Master Teacher, intuitive guide, grief educator, and consciousness explorer with close to three decades of experience in mental health and healing arts. I've supported thousands of people in transforming pain into purpose by bridging the worlds of science and spirit.

As the founder of Hannah's Healing Wellness Studio and co-founder of Path 11 Productions, I've spent over 26 years exploring how energy, frequency, and consciousness shape our emotional and physical well-being. My work blends grounded psychotherapy with energy medicine, sound healing, and spiritually informed techniques that help clients heal their mind, body, and soul.

Whether you're moving through grief, searching for meaning after loss, or simply ready to rise into your highest potential as an entrepreneur, my mission is to help you remember who you really are. I'm ready to guide you to grow and glow as you reclaim your inner light.

When I'm not holding space for healing, you'll find me behind a camera exploring stories of consciousness, leading grief and wellness retreats, or teaching students how to tune their energy to the *I AM* frequency.

If your soul is ready for transformation, visit my link below to begin your *I AM* journey and join my *I AM* Circle membership for extra support throughout the month.

CONNECT WITH APRIL:

LinkTree: https://linktr.ee/AprilAnneHannah

Choosing a modality clashing with personality, beliefs, or subconscious patterns can curdle even the best intentions. When the flavor doesn't fit, we quit the cup—spinning dizzy again in the loop-de-loop of not-enoughness—even mind-whipping ourselves with frothy give-up guilt.

~ Sensei Timothy Stuetz

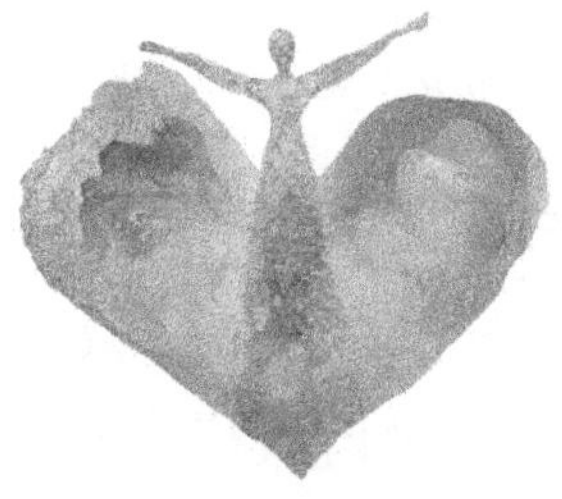

CHAPTER 22

SELF-HEALING'S ANCIENT SECRET SAUCE
NO POTIONS-PROPS-POSITIONS-MOOLAH-MOTIONS-TICK-TOCKS

Sensei Timothy Stuetz

A Secret
So simple—Soul saucy,
Life's linguini twirls to ecstasy!

MT STORY

Being Here
Now is sacred, even
When *Here* is sitt'n bare on toilet throne!

Sitt'n on the deck of the commode,
Wonder'n why it's so hard to dump.
Sitt'n on the deck of the commode,
Feel'n uneasy about this speed bump.
Sitt'n on the deck of the commode,
Things weren't work'n like they should.

Sitt'n on this seat so long can't be good.

Didn't know what good could even be,
Or good was far beyond body harmony.

Who to see, where to go,
To find what I don't yet know?

My self-heal'n quest begins sitt'n on the deck of the commode.

I open the door, leaving the super clean, organically stocked, tastefully and colorfully decorated bathroom of my favorite coffee and cacao café.

Life resumes—
Buzz, beans, banter, and me
Seem'n like I've got it all together.

Wonder'ns and feel'ns of moments past, flush away as coffee and cacao aromas arise.

Choices, so many choices!

Choices delighting my eyes, tantalizing my taste buds, swirling up my nose, soothing my entire being.

Which espresso? Which cacao combination?

I want the best!

It's the same as I write here and now.

Which self-healing practice of the 100+ I know, practice, and am lineage-initiated to teach will instantly and perpetually harmonize and energize your entire being?

What follows isn't just another technique—it's the Ancient Secret Sauce of Self-healing, shaping my bathroom blues into bedtime bliss and me into the sound of one hand clapping.

Lost for centuries—not a product, potion, or prescription—a precious pearlescent pearl to treasure.

A secret you could not use up in a whole lifetime. What more could I teach you?

It's so simple, most folks, hopefully not you, will overlook it, continuing to search for miracles more modern, flashy, and costly.

Sometimes the grandest revelations arise from the humblest seats.

My spontaneous wonder'n while sitt'n on the deck of the commode led me to approach a fellow board member of a Youth-At-Risk network.

Why did I choose Cliff, whom I didn't know?

He's an Aikido Master Teacher, looks in great shape, speaks with conviction, and exudes peace.

Cliff recommends his iridologist.

What's that?

Following her microscopic look into each eye:

What do you mean my body's in such dire straits I need to switch cold turkey to foods, fresh juice combos (some quite nasty), and herbs unknown and foreign to my body terrain?

Talk about a detox crisis and bathroom blues!

Life crisis follows. Far more than my body falls apart—career, marriage, beliefs—life as I knew it.

More self-healing blessings, previously unknown to me, appear.

- Regression, rebirthing

- Hatha yoga

- Siddha yoga meditation

- Reiki

- Massage forms

- Qigong, t'ai chi

- Sound healing

- Medical intuitive training

- Science of Mind ministry

- Reconnecting with Christ

- A transformational ecstasy experience

- Devouring hundreds of spiritual, healing, reincarnation, mind development, visualization, and nutrition books.

Soul blessed,
Each transforms—sheer, tiny
Fraction of known—takes but one koan.

Pile on man-made modalities, and the kaleidoscope of choices twirls one dizzier than spinning on a playground merry-go-round.

Just as people's taste buds differ—one savoring peppermint-cacao, another vanilla-orange; one loving espresso, another a foamy latte—our inner natures crave different healing blends.

Choosing a modality clashing with personality, beliefs, or subconscious patterns can curdle even the best intentions.

When the flavor doesn't fit, we quit the cup—spinning dizzy again in the loop-de-loop of not-enoughness—even mind-whipping ourselves with frothy give-up guilt.

Curious?
Perplexed are you, reading,
Self-healing book, searching for something—

Anything,
Unveiling true essence—
Your body-mind-heart-soulful God Self?

We're like goldfish swimming round 'n round in a glass bowl—searching for freedom.

How curiously crazy to find ourselves doing something, anything, to return to our natural state of peace, love, bliss, and vitality.

All craziness prized—wonder'n how surprised you'll be, discover'n the something sought—

- **Is free,** beyond enjoyable, and longer lasting than any cacao and coffee concoctions we savor.

- Helps you live **pain and thought-free** in blissful ecstasy—an ongoing experience, not a temporary high.

- Requires **no extra time!** No need to forsake anything or squeeze it into an already packed, sardine-tight schedule.

- Is **easy-peasy enjoyable** anywhere, everywhere, any time.

- **Harmonizes** whatever ails, regardless of nature, intensity, duration, your age, and current condition.

- Is as close as your breath, sits on the tip of your tongue, **waits to be savored** like your favorite sunset, dessert, or hugging arms.

And how fantastical would it be if there were several *somethings*—several solutions used for thousands of years in cultures around the world—purringly paired like cacao and coffee, whipped cream and pumpkin pie, waffle cones and ice cream?

Solutions I've practiced and shared for over 44 years with thousands like you, many traumatized beyond imagination.

Whether sitt'n on the deck of the commode, dock of the bay, atop a bale of hay, or searching for something previously as elusive as the proverbial needle in a haystack, your innate wisdom led you to this *Self-Healing Ancient Secret Sauce*—so saucy, soul simple.

What's more, your search ends here, should you so choose.

Ripe to move
Beyond what you're used to—
No matter the discomfort it's caused?

Do you have
Eyes to see, ears to hear,
Heart-speak true, mind and will to follow?

Claim relief,
So endless, so saucy,
So—body, mind, heart, and soul—soothing!

Paramahamsa Yogananda, great master and author of *Autobiography of a Yogi,* asks: "What is it that will destroy pain and ignorance forever, so that your body, mind, and soul will reflect the perfect image of Spirit? It is this: Convince your mind that all human methods of cure are limited in their healing power and that only God's all-permeating healing power is unlimited."

Accessing this unlimited healing power is easy—steadily repeat a mantra—any God-aligned word, phrase. This silent, sacred science convinces, transforms your mind—especially when empowered by a living Master or lineage.

Having any mind qualms?

You can quell them by reading the undeniable, millennial evidence in Chapter #18, "Mantra Momentum Mojo: Believe It, Fake It, Feel It, Become It" in *Expressive Arts: The Ultimate Creative Guide to Transforming Stress* by Jean Voice Dart.

"Mantra Momentum Mojo" is a poetic magic carpet ride on the science, miracles, and benefits of mantra repetition (japa), including my most unfathomable healing experiences—waking, dreaming, meditating.

Japa is nondenominational, universal, appearing throughout traditions worldwide as—

- Om

- Hamsa

- Yod Hey Wah Hey

- Om Namah Shivaya

- I AM Light (or Love or Bliss)

- Christ (or any great being) and I Are One

Thousands there are—Japa's miraculously magical miracle pills.

Relief may be instantaneous or not. Japa doesn't gloss over pain, discomfort, disconnection—*it gets to the roots.*

My adult body's felt insufferable, excruciating pain three times—pain so intense, I wanted to die. Japa saved me. Most recently—November 2022.

I'm sitting in my favorite winter lunch spot overlooking the Mediterranean.

Ahh, soul heavenly. Golden sheen sparkles on the Sea. Sun rays kiss, warming my face.

Suddenly, I'm scripted into a Vietnam movie scene. A black helicopter rises over the nearest hill, whirling toward me.

I watch, frozen in surprise, no clue I'd been locked in. No clue, no time to engage energy shields.

I feel a slight twinge as it passes over.

Hmmm?

Within hours, I'm bedridden—**PAIN** gradually intensifying until excruciating beyond excruciating.

Can't move an inch without ***scroaning***—screaming or groaning—pain flames flaring like gas poured on a fire.

Om. . .Om. . .Om. . .for twelve unbearable, reletless hours before blessed sleep ensues.

Two hours later, I awaken—blissfully pain-free.

Om. . .Om. . .Om. . .Thank You, God!

Om, om, om,
Om, om, om, om, om, om,
God's Roto-Rooter Pain Remover.

Hold on to
Om like super glue bonds,
Repeat *Om* often, every breath!

Yes, there's no
Malaise so severe, a
Japa tidal wave can't wash clear—*Om!*

Pause,
Touch Your Heart.

Inhale Starshine,
Be!

Exhale, Empty,
Satori Be!

Seven days into being pain-free **but not functional,** still spinning in a loop-de-loop extraordinaire—Japa ongoing, sunbathing with bare feet grounded on Mother Earth for 20-30 minutes a day, eating only easily digestible fruits and veggies—I remember the ancient Nei Gung contemplations learned from my first T'ai Chi Master, Justin Stone, in 1986.

Ready for the crème de la crème—the secret within the secret sauce, the ancient, effortless elixir lost for centuries—bubbl'n within these words, self-healing vibes swirling through the lines?

It's called *Zen-Five*—a distilled slice of Nei Gung!

If Qigong is learning to conduct electricity safely and skillfully, Nei Gung is becoming the power plant itself.

Qigong moves energy with ease; Nei Gung's energy *moves the practitioner*—like japa in harmonic overdrive!

Prismatic contemplations crafted for the mind ready to laugh, drift, and awaken all at once—turning subtle energies into physical vitality and full-spectrum awareness.

Light within
Bends, silent truth angles
Refract, colorful stillness ensues.

Pre-internet and AI, Justin discovered Zen Master Hakuin's first four *Tanden Contemplations* (hereafter called Zen-Four) in a book falling on him from a jam-packed shelf along the narrow aisles of a bookstore, dusty antiquity permeating the air.

Justin taught them as *Nei Gung* (hereafter called Stone's-Four) during my Seijaku training.

Still within,
Center moves, yet unmoved,
Alive, flowing—mind, heart wide open.

I practice *Stone's-Four* nightly—lying down, as recommended, before going to sleep. Immediately, sleep ensues faster and deeper than ever, forever—for which they are renowned.

Six months later, I commit to repeating them until a dynamic experience arises—even if it means an all-nighter!

Why?

Because Justin **said** Master Hakuin used nothing but Stone's-Four in his late twenties to not only cure his emotional and physical health, which had seriously deteriorated to the point where he was ready to leave his body—*Zen Meditation Sickness*—but to enlighten him in the process.

My soul whispers: *Me too!*

After about 30 minutes of repetition, every cell of my body ignites like a glowing SUN.

I'm sparkling—every pore shining bright!

My senses soar. I'm hearing, clear as whispers in my ear, conversations and noises in distant parts of the house, behind walls and closed doors, as well as outside, as far away as across the street.

Nothing but ecstasy beyond ecstasy I AM!

Since this knock-my-socks-off extravaganza, I only use this kaleidoscopic *Stone's-Four* when I feel physically wiped out or super stuck, needing a breakthrough—and grace faithfully moves through.

Stone's-Four—I
Turn, trust, test, then hit it—
Kaleidoscopic jackpot, sage shifts.

Jackpot for me, Mega Lottery for you—*KA-POW!*

While penning
This prose, whispers I hear—
Research *Stone's-Four story, not questioned.*

Truth revealed—
Hakuin, not yet age
Thirty, near death, Zen O.D., seeks help.

Treks to cave,
High in mountains, home of
Hakuyu—age, three hundred plus years.

Remedies—
See soft butter melting,
Head to soles through body, feel the glow.

Belly breaths,
Tanden focus too. **No**
Stone's-Four in Hakuin's self-healing.

Hakuin,
Koan ace, ten years hence,
Births *Zen-Four.* More years pass—*Fifth* evolves.

Tanden to
Soles, energy sea flows.
Fivefold tide turns form—formless; blues—bliss.

Stone finds four,
Silently fine tunes tone,
Zen-Four matures to thunderous roar.

Hakuyu—
Seed. Hakuin—garden.
Stone—hybridizer. Stuetz—*Full Lotus*.

Lineage
Revered—Stone's facelift flow,
Hakuin's Fifth, with grand *Zen-Five* twist.

Yes, you get
The full *Zen-Five* Monty,
Secret sauce stewed seven centuries.

And while *Om* dissolved all pain, I'm still reeling, wiped out, needing another breakthrough.

The number of *Stone's-Four* super-healing, prismatic contemplations repeated before falling asleep, I know not.

On returning to consciousness around 5 a.m., I'm feeling embraced in the afterglow of a satsang—like I've been chanting and meditating with my spiritual family since falling asleep.

This is soul wonderful, peaceful, fantastical. I want to bring all my friends, family, students, and everyone I've ever met to be with me in and as this peaceful bliss.

Amidst this desire, I fall back asleep.

Several hours later, waking consciousness returns—only the me who dozed back to sleep was not there.

Awaken
As *nothing,* God's pure love,
Mind-blown, heart-full, bliss-full without end!

Body lying in bed, *I AM pulsating atoms of God's pure love.*

I don't want to move or do anything else, ever!

I AM complete.

I don't want to ever lose this feeling, this awareness—this beingness and yet nothingness!

I melt back to sleep in this bliss-beyond-bliss for just a bit before arising.

Body feels
Like when first fell asleep,
Yet awareness remains—God's pure love.

Another Stone's-Four breakthrough beyond imaginable!

With most of what was left of the Timothy I knew obliterated, I moved about all day in blessed and blissful beingness.

The physical imbalances and lack of energy continued, but I experienced a *wholly, holy,* different state mentally, emotionally, and as simply being.

God's grace, soul amazing, coupled with my will to repeat *Stone's-Four* once again—just like decades before with my first all-nighter commitment—created another unexpected miracle.

A week later, still transformed in every way—but physically—the blessings of continuing Stone's-Four repetitions nightly again weaved their magic.

Twas a night inundated with one weird, crazy vivid dream after another. Very weird and crazy dreams, not my norm, amidst intermittent surges of energy up into my crown chakra—uncomfortably intense at times.

New day dawns, I feel 50% more energetic than when I went to sleep. Physical and mental vitality slowly and steadily increased over the next nine weeks, including the ability to create, write, and walk-up hills to regain my lung power and endurance.

More threads of
What was once Timothy
Dissolved in those dreams, energy swells.

Blessed swells,
Less intense, persist, roll
In nightly, clearing in mystery.

Vim, vigor
Rise daily. Energy
Ascends to levels pre-copter strike.

Small price paid
For karmic blocks busted.
Awareness true, forever redeemed.

Few days pass,
Awake, feeling inner
Bliss and playfulness zapped five weeks past.

Morning next,
Before opening eyes,
Crown shakti surges, lava cresting.

Dream dragons
Come, spewing love flames through
My being—*soul beyond blissed I AM.*

Namaste
Dragon friends, highest love
Bearers, foreseers beyond all realms.

Namaste
Bookworm friend—Curious
Are you about this poetic style?

Bonus-tool,
Vibrational blessings,
You can scribe too—miracles ensue.

3:6:9
Code, so magnificent.
It holds keys to Universe—unlock!

Tesla Threes,
Harmonic harmonies,
Lines uniting mind, body, heart, soul.

Syllables,
Line one, 3; Line two, 6;
Line three, 9. Now, it's versify time.

Tesla Tiers,
Stack lines three, story grows.
Three, six, nine stanzas—ready-set-GO!

Choose your words,
Let them bloom—love notes, memes,
Affirmations, logos, ads, posts, books.

Potent force,
They design. Strong, they are.
Language they shape, children's minds they guide.

All our minds,
Poetic pep pills pure.
Tesla Tyme Poems—shift lives, shape worlds.

Self-healing
Tools two, your hands now hold.
Japa—*Om,* 3:6:9 soul-u-tions!

Zen-Five's next!
Your Ancient Secret Sauce.
Structure, rhythm, resonance—MU's might—POW!

Just a pause,
Bathroom bare, led me here,
Sitt'n on a Gold *Zen-Five* Toilet Throne.

Pause,
Touch Your Heart.

Breathe,
Soften,
Be *Om!*

Now, let's get you—

Sitt'n on the deck of enlightened living,
Sail'n downwind—beyond health, peace 'n loving.
Sitt'n on the deck of enlightened living,
Feel'n groovy with everything aligning.

Sitt'n on the deck of enlightened living,
Everything humm'n in tune, beyond imagining.

Let's get you—

Sitt'n on this soul-song seat, blissfully free.
Know'n what living in ecstasy can be,
It's soul way beyond body harmony.
Sitt'n on the deck of enlightened living,
Nowhere to go now—you are *the Tao,*
Relax'n into living, *being here now.*

Hakuyu,
Hakuin, Stone, Sensei Stuetz—
Tone, Lyrics, Harmony, Resonance.

Take your seat,
Zen Symphony—*Stone's-Four,*
Hakuin's Fifth, with grand *Zen-Five* twist.

Our hands to
Yours, healing vibes pass on—
Zen-Five echoes—timeless One Hand sound.

THE TOOL

ZEN-FIVE, SECRET SAUCE RECIPE!

Power up. Connect within—your lineage bona fide.

Hold intention: *This is my miraculous secret sauce—unimaginable wonders incoming.*

Lying down or sitting comfortably, legs gently pressed together, repeat the contemplations—*awareness flows like breath following light*—tracing your words from the *tanden* (two finger widths below the navel) to the *soles of your feet,* life's bubbl'n springs.

With repetition, the contemplations memorize themselves—*not as something you do—but becoming what moves through and as you.*

REFRAIN-BEGINS EACH CONTEMPLATION:

This Energy Sea, this tanden, from below the navel to the soles of the feet—

CONTEMPLATIONS-SEQUENCE TRUE:

- Full of my Original Face. *Where are the nostrils on that Face?*

- Full of my True Home. *What need of a message from that Home?*

- Full of the Pure Land of Consciousness only. *What need of outer pomp has this Pure Land?*

- Full of the Amida Buddha of heart and body. *What sermon would this Amida be preaching?*

- Full of Mu (pronounced moo)—emptiness alive, nothing that's everything. *What is the sound of one hand clapping?*

Paraphrasing Buddha

He who keeps his concentration in the
soles of his feet will heal 1000 illnesses.

Prior to transitioning at age 90, Taiwanese Master Liu of T'ai Chi Gik—

Science rare,
Seasonal touch through time,
Master's yin-yang, tap-strike, heals or slays

offered Justin this enhancement on *Stone's-Four*—

"For those who have the privacy: lay nude on the Earth, facing up to the sun, taking in the *yang* (positive) of the sun and absorb the *yin* (negative) of the Earth at the same time."

And Hakuin (January 19, 1686 - January 18, 1769),
nearing his final breath, pens:

An elderly monk of eighty-four, I welcome in yet one more year
And I owe it all—everything—to the Sound of One Hand barrier.

Our hands to

Yours, healing vibes pass on—
Zen-Five echoes—timeless One Hand sound.

Aerated,
This secret sauce word count—
Three-thousand-**six**—sum **nine**—*KaPow!*

Your *Zen-Five* Mega Lottery Loot—

- Secret Sauce Contemplation Audio—**30:06** minutes—Cosmic Choreography

- Two High-Five songs

- *Zen-Five* Deep Dive

- Secret-Saucey Surprise

Click. Breathe. Be Mu.

Savor your saucy *Zen-Five secret sauce* today—
3:6:9—GO! https://www.timothystuetz.com/zen-five

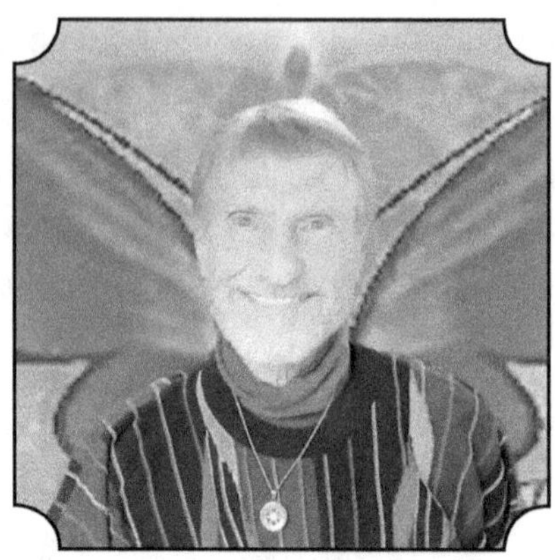

"Self-Healing
Climax—pierce ego's veils—
Embody, thrive, live as your God-Self!"

Sensei Timothy, **The Magical & Mystical Fairy Tale Wizard & Poet** is a visionary educator, celebrated for writing 90+ songs and 290+ children's stories—100+ more than Hans Christian Andersen.

For over four decades, he's woven **fairy tales, meditation, Reiki, qigong, yoga, and everything in between,** empowering thousands—from Bali to Cali—to remember and use Source powers to achieve their full potential.

A Science of Mind Minister, Retired CPA, Amazon #1 bestselling author, and Book Excellence Award Winner, he consciously weaves **myth and mystery, fantasy and reality, poetry and proven human development principles** to ignite creativity, vitality, bliss, brilliance—wiring everyone for success.

He's created:

- **BE: Blissfully Empowered**—a 1:1, 12-month personalized transformation with 24/7 support.

- **Bliss Weaving Community Circle**—four 90-minute group sessions monthly.

- **Sacred Sciences Alchemy Academy**—turning teens and adults into *Certified Personal & Business Black Belts.*

- **Bliss Beary Bears Be-Yond-A Book Club**—including weekly live story times and bi-weekly parent circles.

- **The Magical Miracle of You**—a children's and family self-development program.

- **Tesla 3:6:9 Personal Empowerment Poems.**

Embracing souls at birth, death, and through challenges colossal and minute, he lives within an ever-unfolding miracle:

- Seeing crystalline white light as the screen God's many faces play on.

- Enjoying a patient, serene, steady mind.

- Feeling Universal Energy pulse through his body—strong, flexible, and medication free.

- Laughing freely, sparked solely and soulfully within.

- Immersed in harmonic inner music and the sacred silence from which all sounds arise.

- Free of fear, addiction, anger, and despair.

All his creations are shaped by **Grace** and **75+ years of wonders**—including the humbling, heart-opening adventure of being a father.

Connect with Timothy:

Website: https://www.timothystuetz.com

Email: timothy@timothystuetz.com

Linktr.ee: https://linktr.ee/timothystuetz.com

Self-healing begins on a pathway to peace and calm, where presence, breath, and stillness become medicine.

~ Brigette Burton

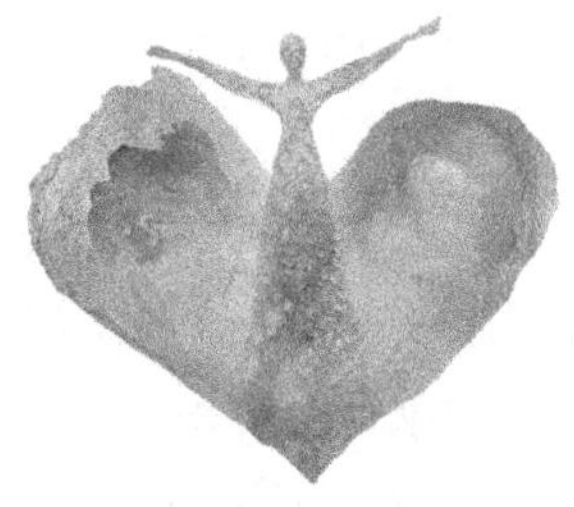

CHAPTER 23

A Pathway to Calm and Peace
Mind-Body Connection

Brigette Burton

Author, Poet, Mental Health Advocate

"Self-healing begins on a pathway to peace and calm, where presence, breath, and stillness become medicine."
~Brigette Burton

My Story

Entrance Into the World of Calm

"Brigette, will you start and find the first two words: a-b-u-n-d-a-n-t-l-y and d-e-d-i-c-a-t-i-o-n, for your group?"

I barely heard the question. My body sank into the plastic seat, my head hidden between two books to avoid attention. My lungs clung tight beneath the invisible weight of anxiety. It felt like an elephant curled up on my chest, each breath tangled in the clutter of mental exhaustion. My thoughts collided like bumper cars; my neurons fired in frantic loops.

But then—something shifted.

I sat up slowly, almost involuntarily, and scanned the Seek-n-Find puzzle sheet lying face down on the desk. Within seconds, the two words emerged like stars breaking through thick fog. "Wow, you're fast," the teacher said. Her voice tinged with surprise. "How'd you find the two words so quickly?"

I wanted to answer, to explain how the chaos in my mind momentarily cleared, how the act of searching for those words soothed something deep inside me. But shyness held my voice hostage. In my mind, I held the strategies I used to bring the words straight into view. I didn't have to search. They were already sitting there, waiting for me to check off.

"Say something."

"Explain. Don't freeze."

"They won't understand unless you speak."

These thoughts surged through my mind like a tide against a sealed door—pressing, pulsing, begging me to let them in.

In that moment, I learned that when the brain is locked in confusion and fear, a simple puzzle can become a key to unlocking clarity, clearing cluttered cells, calming the storm, and guiding the neurons back to a peaceful state. From that day forward, puzzles became my forever partner. I didn't just solve them—I lived in them. They became my address, my solace, a way of protecting myself from waves of doubt, fear, and uncertainty trying to take over.

Every store I entered—grocery stores, department stores, bookstores, thrift shops—I scanned the aisles for puzzles, purchasing them in bulk in all shapes and sizes.

I coated my mind with two quiet strategies—tools that helped me find the words quickly, and more importantly, helped me locate pieces of myself. I always told myself that I'd share and help others learn puzzling strategies to promote joy and happiness.

PUZZELING THROUGH LIFE:
HEALING MINDS, ONE PAGE, ONE LETTER AT A TIME

As I grew older, puzzles followed me like a loyal companion. In classrooms, they became my teaching tool. In workshops, they were my bridge to connection. With clients—stroke survivors, heart attack patients, cancer patients, children with autism—they became my medicine for wellness.

Three to four days a week, sometimes through the weekend, I sat with a close client who was recovering from two strokes. His speech slurred from the strokes, his face was always tight with frustration, his voice sharp with anger and disbelief.

The client asked, "Why do you come here with a bag of puzzle books all the time?"

"I love puzzles," I replied. "They're fun, challenging, and really great for sharpening my brain. They keep me busy, happy, focused, and calm."

"That's crazy!" he said, with a stale look on his face. "How in the world can puzzles make you happy? There's no way a puzzle can calm me down or make me happy. With all this stuff going on with me, I don't have time to think about anything but what I'm going through. I'm sick of this mess."

I placed my hand atop his, smiled gently, letting his words settle in the space between us.

"I hear you," I said softly. "Hey, but what if we just try it out, not try to solve the whole thing? What if we play and see how you feel afterwards?" I suggested.

He raised his eyebrows and hand. "Play?" he asked in a deep tone.

"Yes," I said. "Let's play one-on-one. Set the timer. Race the clock. Let the puzzle be the challenge—not your body, not your mind. Just the puzzle." He hesitated, gave a heavy sigh, then nodded. I handed him a seek-and-find sheet and clicked the timer.

"Ready? Go!"

At first, he grumbled through a few visits. His arms folded tight across his chest, his eyes darting toward the clock more than the puzzle sheets. The frustration sat heavy in the room, like fog that refused to lift. I didn't push. I laid out the puzzles—Sudoku, crosswords, Seek 'n' Find, logic games—and invited him to play.

By the third visit, he was different. It was like his aura gave a sense of freedom, releasing him from a makeshift cell.

He waited at the door before I could even unpack my bags. "You got that number one puzzle again?" he asked, voice still gruff but tinged with curiosity. "The one with the boxes and the numbers?"

"Sudoku?" I smiled.

"Yeah, that one. I want to beat the timer with this one, then race against you with another seek-and-find puzzle."

"Well, now look at this. I love the enthusiasm. Let's do it," I replied.

I handed him the sheet and clicked the stopwatch. His fingers moved faster now, his brow furrowed in focus, not in frustration. The puzzle became a challenge, not a chore. A spark lit behind his eyes, something I had never seen before.

Then came a moment that changed everything completely.

I introduced him to my two favorite game shows: *Wheel of Fortune* and *Jeopardy.* "You ever watch this?" I asked as I turned on the TV.

The client shrugged. "I used to. Back when things were better," he said, with his voice hurried and grumpy.

We sat together, side by side, as letters flipped and the wheel spun. We raced against each other, trying to solve the puzzles before the buzzer. When we blurted out the wrong answers, he burst into laughter—deep, belly-shaking laughter that brought tears to his eyes.

"Oh man," he said, wiping his face. "I can't believe I missed that one! I was off by one word."

The change was remarkable. His speech improved, and the tight knot in his shoulders released.

From here, he made sure we sat in front of the television by 7:00 p.m. sharp. "Don't be late," he said. "I got big guesses in me tonight."

He looked forward to the puzzles. He asked about new ones. He wanted to try harder ones. He even started creating his own clues. I watched in awe, my heart full of joy.

The transformation wasn't just cognitive—it was emotional, spiritual, and relational. The puzzles became a bridge, a balm, a way back to himself. I felt good inside seeing him happy.

In classrooms, children began to light up when the timer buzzed. Their giggles spread across the room. They pointed and shouted out words. I saw how their bodies relaxed, how their eyes sparkled, how their little minds, once tangled in sensory overload, found rhythm in the structure of play.

Noticing the shift in brainwaves, I found it essential to carry puzzles into places where pain and sorrow lived loudly—battered women's shelters, barbershops filled with quiet tension, senior homes where silence hung heavy, and youth centers where teens wore armor made of sarcasm and side eyes. I didn't come with answers. I came with puzzles.

At first, the answers were predictable.

"I don't do puzzles. That's for kids," some teens would say." "I'm too tired to play," some would yell out.

But I smiled and said, "Come on, just five minutes. Let's race the timer. You'll have fun. Let's try it." After getting them to connect, it was easy from there. They rushed to their favorite chairs, ready for the challenge. It was like playing musical chairs when they saw me coming.

In a shelter, a woman who hadn't spoken in days whispered, "I found the word freedom." Her fingers trembled as she pointed to the page. Her smile spread loosely across her face. We all paused. That word became a prayer. She appeared vibrant, surprised, and energetic. The act of working that puzzle made a big difference.

In the barbershops where I dropped off some of my tasty cakes, men who usually debated sports and politics began competing over crossword clues. One man shouted, "Hey man, I got the word r-e-s-i-l-i-e-n-c-e—beat that!" The room erupted in laughter and peaceful chatter. The puzzles softened the edges in the shared environment.

At the senior home, one resident refused to play. "My mind's too old for this mess," she blurted out. But after watching others laugh and cheer, she joined in. By the end of the week, she led the puzzle circle, glasses perched on her nose, calling out clues like a game show host. I was amazed by the shift in her attitude.

Teenagers, skeptical and guarded, started asking, "You got any new ones today, Ms. BB?" They began to look forward to the challenge. Their moods calmed, their posture changed. Their eyes lit up. Seeing their bodies connect with their thoughts was amazing. The puzzles didn't fix everything. But they cracked open the door to joy.

MY MOTHER'S LOVE FOR SCRABBLE

"I'm sorry, but your mother has multiple myeloma. It's a rare type of skin cancer representing about one point eight percent of all new cancer cases. I want to schedule her for a biopsy." It was hard hearing the doctors deliver the news, watching my mother's head drop into her lap afterwards. It was a hard pill to swallow, and one of the hardest days of my life. But it didn't keep her away from two of her favorite buddies: Crossword puzzles and Scrabble.

"Yes, Mom. We'd love to play." My sisters and I burst into laughter. A laugh that had our stomachs in pain—she had the game already laid out on the table, ahead of asking if we wanted to join.

Scrabble wasn't just a weekend of fun and pleasure—it was our family's bonding time—a time to bask in each other's worlds. The board appeared on Friday evening like a sacred altar, with time running over into the next morning at times. By Sunday night, we'd still be spelling out laughter and legacy. Sometimes, the game spilled into the week, tiles scattered across the table like breadcrumbs leading us back to each other. My mother's love for puzzles was like sunlight through a storm—steady, warm, and always reaching for joy, even when pain tried to dim the room.

Her love for them deepened during her cancer diagnosis. Scrabble was quality time and a source of happy moments together. We gathered around the table from sunup to sundown, battling for the highest score, the largest word, the title of Scrabble Queen. My youngest sister always dominated the score and took the title until one day, my eldest sister beat her. With my youngest sister's competitive spirit, she was unable to accept the defeat. To our surprise, she flipped the board, preventing us from seeing the final scores. Tiles flew across the table like a force of wind scattering leaves across lawns. Some landed in the kitchen, others landed in the living room.

My mom shook her head with laughter, her face turned up in disbelief. But it didn't stop her from wanting to play another game.

The chemo sessions couldn't even hold her down. When her body ached and energy waned, she still managed to say, "Let's play Scrabble." We saw how tired she was and begged her to rest. "Just one round," she'd insist. Her fingers hovered over the tiles like a chess master scanning the board with fierce determination—calculating, remembering, ready to strike and politely yell, "Checkmate!"

One day, near the end, when she fell weaker from the symptoms, she sat at the table, pain etched into every line of her face. We asked, "Mom, why don't you lie down for a while?" She disregarded our plea.

She nodded off mid-turn, tiles clutched in her hand. We gently woke her, and through the haze of pain, she chuckled hard and blurted, "I'm not asleep—I have my word right here!"

My sisters and I laughed until our faces were wet with tears, until our bellies were in knots. Between the hurt and sadness, the moment became a treasure, a memory we never forgot.

Scrabble gave her something to hold onto. She went from Scrabble to scrambling through her piles of crossword puzzles. It shifted her brainwaves from suffering to joy, from pain to play. It was more than a game; it was a lifeline.

Even in her final days, at times, she chose letters over silence and laughter over despair. Her legacy lives in every puzzle I share, every word I help someone find.

Because sometimes, the simplest puzzle can become the most potent medicine—a natural cure for mental strain.

THE SCIENCE OF JOY FOUND IN PUZZLE PIECES

Here's what I found happening beneath the surface of working through puzzles—not just in behavior, but in the brain itself.

Puzzling shifts neuro-chemicals. It nudges the brain toward the release of dopamine—the joy chemical. It overrides the negative neurons, quiets the angry and frustrated ones. Working puzzles isn't just for pleasure; it's a biological override. It's not just a distraction, it's a transformation.

When someone completes a puzzle, even a small one, the brain registers a sense of success. That success sends a signal: *You're safe. You're capable. You're here.* And in that moment, the negative neurons—the ones wired for stress, fear, or fatigue—quiet down.

Clients reported sleeping better and experiencing less anxiety, laughing more, and feeling lighter—their bodies relaxed with less tension. Their moods lifted. Their minds and bodies connected in ways that felt unfamiliar, yet sincerely welcome. These are feelings traditional therapy couldn't reach.

One client said, "Wow, I feel like my brain got a message. I feel different."

Another whispered, "I didn't think I could feel joy again. But I do, now. Thank you so much."

What they were experiencing wasn't just emotional—it's also neurological. Puzzles activate the prefrontal cortex, the part of the brain responsible for decision-making, focus, and emotional regulation. They also engage the hippocampus, which plays a crucial role in supporting memory and learning. When both areas light up, the body follows: heart rate slows, breath deepens, muscles soften.

It's a full-body shift.

Even the act of searching for a word in word find puzzles, completing a space in crossword puzzles, and using strategy to solve number puzzles like Sudoku creates a rhythmic pattern in the brain, much like a heartbeat.

That rhythm sends calming signals to the nervous system. It's why people feel soothed, even if they aren't able to solve the puzzle.

I've seen this effect become magnified in trauma-informed spaces, and I was the first to witness it through the lens of my own trauma.

Survivors of abuse, grief, or some illness often carry hyper-vigilant nervous systems. But when they engage with puzzles, their parasympathetic system—the "rest and digest" mode—activates. Their bodies begin to trust the moment. Their minds start to breathe.

Puzzles don't just entertain; they restore. They remind the brain that joy is possible, that clarity can return, that peace isn't distant; it's near, waiting to soothe.

THE PUZZLE PRESCRIPTION: TAKE TWO PUZZLES AND CALL ME IN THE MORNING

The connection between mind and body is the most important reason I love puzzling so much, and why I love sharing puzzling as a tool, not just a pastime, as a means of healing through mind-mapping.

It's an ultimate pathway to peace and calm—a mind-body connection that doesn't require words, diagnosis, or perfection, just presence—and a natural way to help calm feelings. It leaves a healing impact.

Puzzles don't fix the pain, but they ease and minimize it. They offer a gentle doorway to re-enter the body. This is why I call it a prescription. Not written on paper, but felt in the breath. Not handed out, but invited in.

And now, I invite you into this world of presence. One piece, one page at a time. Enjoy!

THE TOOL

Many people have found their way back to peace through play and problem-solving, not through force or fixing, but through gentle invitation. The puzzle became more than a pastime. It became a prescription, a daily companion, an entry into calm.

Now, I offer it to you—not as a cure-all, but as an arc for healing. A tool to help you breathe deeper, think clearly, and feel more connected to your body's wisdom and brain's connections. It leads to a wealth of healthy thoughts and peaceful moments, even amid waves of darkness, despair, and uncertainty.

Below, you'll find a pathway I've used for decades with humanity, using different methods. Now, I offer you this pathway.

A Guide to Cognitive Health

STEP 1: THE INVITATION

- Ask the client/person, "Would you be willing to play with me for five minutes?"

- Offer a simple puzzle: seek-and-find, wordsearch, crossword, sudoku, or matching game.

STEP 2: TEAM PLAY

- Break into pairs, small groups, or one-on-one play.

- Set a timer for five to ten minutes.

- Celebrate every find with joy and happy feelings.

STEP 3: REFLECTION

- Breathe/Ask: "How did your body feel before and after?"

- Invite the person to name one emotion that shifted.

STEP 4: INTEGRATION

- Suggest a daily puzzle day.

- Encourage framing, posting the completed puzzle, journaling, or drawing after completing

STEP 5: EXPANSION

- Introduce new puzzle types.

- Invite them to create their own puzzles with clues.

GUIDING QUESTIONS:

- What does calm feel like in your body?

- What puzzle made you feel most alive?

- Where in your life could you use more play with puzzles?

I hope you enjoy the tool. And, if you find yourself falling into a dark space, I invite you to return here for comfort.

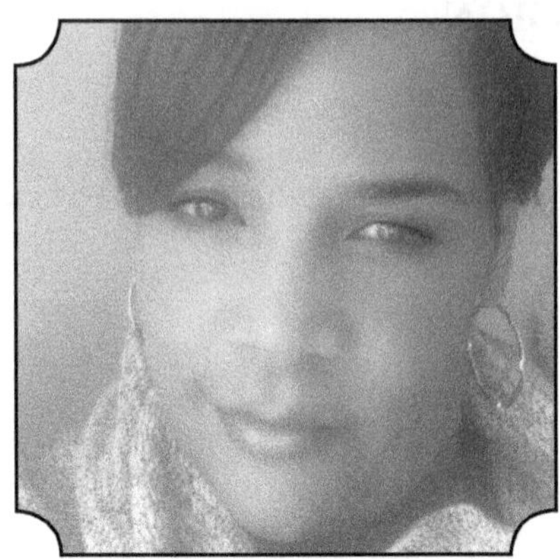

Brigette M. Burton is a best-selling author, poetic healer, and founder of Soul Works Publications—a legacy imprint devoted to transformative storytelling, emotional resilience, mental strengthening, and self-healing practices.

Have you ever sought peace amidst your pain? Walk with Brigette on a pathway to calm and peace, where words become medicine and memory becomes light. Her story, *A Pathway to Calm and Peace: Mind-Body Connection,* invites readers on a journey of mental mapping strategies, caregiving methods, and transformation. Her writing blends neuroscience with lived truth, introducing self-healing practices through creative processes. Brigette guides readers to re-enter their stories with grace. Her work honors the sacred pause, the handwritten voice, and emotional truth that lives beneath the surface.

Brigette facilitates workshops for adults, teens, and children using puzzles, art, music, and poetic therapy to unlock emotional freedom. She is intentional in every detail—curating experience with emotional resonance, symbolic depth, and a focus on growth and inner development rather than technical skill. Her sessions invite participants to explore healing through creative ritual, sensory engagement, and reflective prompts that honor both personal story and collective transformation. Whether guiding a child through watercolor emotions or inviting others to write legacy lines. She creates spaces where vulnerability becomes strength, and expression becomes medicine. Her work is a living embodiment of the mind-body connection—a pathway to peace that begins with presence, creativity, and the courage to feel.

When Brigette takes a break from her writing path, you can find her dancing around with her grandchildren, crafting stories from puzzle pieces, or painting emotions with watercolors and wonder.

For healing that begins at home.

CONNECT WITH BRIGETTE:

Email: bhglitteredsoul6117@gmail.com

Instagram: https://www.instagram.com/legacyoflove5813

Facebook: https://facebook.com/brigetteburton

What if I can change the expression of the traumatic experience? I can't change the actual event, but I can change how my body energetically and emotionally holds it!

~ Laura Mayer

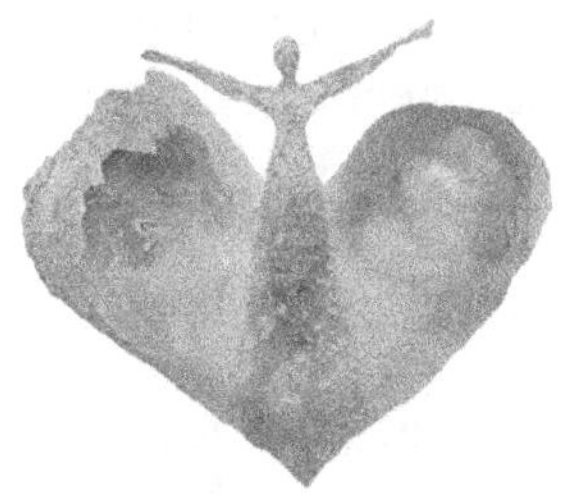

The Transformational Power of Epigenetics
Go to the Core-Heal So Much More

Laura Mayer

M.A., OTR, Epigenetic Therapist

My Story

"You are all about epigenetics."

Those five words changed the course of my life forever.

It's August 2011, and I'm driving to Boston from New York—my heart pounds, filled to the brim with anticipation. I'm going to see my favorite neurologist, Dr. Steve Horowitz, the chief resident in neurology, who performed my EMGs when I was fifteen.

It has been thirty-seven years since I was his patient. Words cannot describe my excitement. I feel the resurgence of my teenage crush.

I wonder if he's still so good-looking.

Is he still so tall?

I am thrilled for him to see me, so many decades later, happy and healthy.

He will be shocked. Laura, just drive!

Dr. Horowitz walks into the medical center lobby, where we agreed to meet. As he approached, I noticed he held a small index card. Lifting it, he said, "This was you at fifteen. Your trajectory was so horrific that I specialized in neurology because of you. I thought you were dead."

He's still tall, still attractive. This is surreal.

He was visibly stunned—not just because I'm alive, but because I'm smiling, vibrant, and thriving.

"I often wondered over the years if you might be dead, as predicted by the Chief of Neurology."

We spent the next two hours catching up as I shared with him the last four decades of my life: fifteen hand surgeries, my opening to the metaphysical field, the profound sadness of saying goodbye to my beloved profession, and my transformation by relentlessly believing I could heal.

When I finished, he looked at me and said,

"You are all about epigenetics."

He explains that epigenetics is a relatively new field in medicine that focuses on our ability to change from a negative state (disease) to a positive state (wellness).

"Have you heard about epigenetics?

"No," I reply.

I sat there trying to absorb what Dr. Horowitz said.

I'm completely immersed in metaphysics and spirituality; the last thing I want to do is dive back into the medical world. I lived there my whole life. Why would I want to return?

Because Dr. Horowitz was my hero of sorts, I listened with an open heart.

ENDINGS AND BEGINNINGS

I feel like a deer in the headlights, always having to be aware of everything my freaking hands do. The good occupational therapist knows professionally what energy expenditure means (how much physical muscle strength to use because it's so important not to overdo), but the audacious woman with a disease says: *Screw you. I'm gonna do it no matter what!*

Although frustrated, I try my utmost to figure things out, stay functional, and complete the task at hand. But reality creeps in every time, and the simple act of sitting at the computer for five minutes stresses my aching arms, just as holding my coffee mug or brushing my daughter's hair does.

After forty years, the disease wins and breaks my heart and spirit. At the age of forty-five, my professional career came to a screeching halt. I knew I didn't have the muscle strength to do everything I needed to do. It's all too much on my diseased body; raising children, being a wife, and working full-time. After fifteen tendon transfers and bone fusions, my hand surgeon gives me a dire warning.

"If you don't stop working, you won't have hands at fifty."

I heeded his advice. *What am I to do? I have young children who need me. They come first.*

I was heartbroken.

What am I supposed to do with my life now?

I'm physically and emotionally exhausted from having little to no hand strength. The dynamometer, a tool used in rehabilitation therapies, measures hand strength. I have zero. A normal woman my age has approximately 65 pounds of muscle strength in her hands.

I have to find something, anything, that will help me keep going.

A few years after my career ended, I took a leap of faith and fully dipped my toes into a spiritual renewal center about 90 minutes from where I lived. There I found comfort, support, and community. Chanting, meditating, and Kabbalistic healing have become my new life. I feel at home.

Through the loss, I silently screamed: *Please give me a better life than the one I was handed.*

I knew my heart was opening to something bigger, though I didn't know yet what that meant.

One day, just hanging out at the renewal center, a practitioner of Jin Shin Jyutsu asked, "Can I do a session with you?" He is curious to see if he can help my ailing hands. After the session, he recommended I continue. "I know healing will happen."

Of course, I'll continue. What do I have to lose?

A NEW PAGE

Jed, the practitioner, is located in Woodstock, New York, about an hour and a half from my home. I love Woodstock, and happily made the trek to see what would unfold. After the sixth session, he shared, "You have a profound transformation ahead," and recommended I see a medical intuitive.

Shortly after this last session with Jed, I experienced a profound sense of loss and sadness; I stood in my living room, looking out my side glass door. I felt a sense of doom, as if there was nowhere for me to go.

I feel like I'm riddled with bone cancer. How am I going to survive this disease for another forty years?

It is ten days shy of my fiftieth birthday.

I called the medical intuitive Jed recommended and made an appointment.

And then, just like following the Hansel and Gretel path of bread crumbs, one profound healer after another enters my path.

Am I Gretel? What else can I do but leap into the world of metaphysics and alternative healing?

Filled with despair for my life and hope for a miracle, I opened wide to intuitive readings and energetic healing. I spent hours every day reading books on esoteric healing from various perspectives, including Buddhist, Hindu, Sufi, mystical Kabbalah, and Hebrew teachings.

For the next fifteen years, I heard the same message from every practitioner I saw that surely trumps the devastating diagnosis I received from the medical world:

You will completely heal.

I literally and figuratively have nothing to lose.

WHAT DO I HAVE TO LOSE?

I knew from clinical experience and personal history that there are no quick fixes, such as surgery or pills, that could restore muscle strength and function. I also knew I didn't have the time to engage in spiritual bypassing. Who has time for that?

I did something most would be afraid of; I opened myself to a belief system I know nothing about.

I believe this deep within: if I can heal my heart, my physical body can heal. The funny thing is that at the time, I had no clue that the hands and heart are in the same chakra.

I still get a chuckle from that. With this intention, I immerse myself fully. I'm not the person to fake it until I make it.

Instead, I coach myself: *Stay grounded. Do the work. Remember, there's no "La La Land" when survival is at stake.*

Every morning, I stood in front of my huge bedroom windows and lovingly stroked my hands one at a time.

I proclaimed, "I love you, I love you," as I stretched open my clawed, curled fingers, one hand at a time, both hands in motion, loving each one to wellness with grace and an open heart.

Positive thoughts and energy will heal my hands.

After a year and a half of this practice, my fingers open, one finger at a time. *I know if I love my hands, they will love me back.*

I made a deliberate choice to delay my yearly visit to my hand surgeon until each finger was straight. Once again, with a heart full of awe and joy, I took the familiar route along the Massachusetts Turnpike to Boston to see another doctor, this time, my hand surgeon.

I walk into Mark's office. I've known him for almost thirty years.

It's been two years since my last annual visit. I keep my hands in my lap until he walks in.

He enters the room, hugs me, sits down to examine me, and says, "How are you? It's been a while!"

I lift my hands off my lap and show him my straight fingers. Bewildered, he says, "You are a miracle! Whatever you are doing, keep doing it."

"Mark, I am not a miracle. I stepped into something I knew nothing about! That is where miracles happen."

And miracles did happen!

Over the course of two years, I witnessed profound healing and transformation, and I'm slowly regaining hand function.

Overwhelming joy radiates throughout my entire body every time I pick up my coffee mug singlehandedly or open a jar.

So many tasks—the ones that hurt and the impossible ones—I begin to do. My heart continues to open to a place I didn't know was possible.

I am living proof that healing happens. "Proof is in the pudding" becomes my new motto.

I embody the words of Louise Hay, *You Can Do It,* and Dr. Bruce Lipton, *Change Your Beliefs, Change Your Biology.* I'm on a mission to do just that.

I feel my heart and spirit returning!

It's exhilarating to watch my hands engage in activities I couldn't do for decades.

I have no idea that another equally huge piece of healing was yet to be revealed.

Door Opening

Eight years after I met with Dr. Horowitz, the words clicked. "You are all about epigenetics!"

My eyes opened wide.

My mother is in a coma. She had a cardiac arrest. My sister called the EMTs, and they revived her just long enough to give me time to heal on an entirely different level.

I sat beside her. She was frozen, then warmed. The medical world tells me that's protocol.

We waited to see if she had any brain functioning.

I sang and spoke lovingly and tenderly. For me, this time with her is a gift from the Universe.

I showed up with grace and gratitude.

The softness was palpable between my mother and me. I cherish the moments I have, knowing clearly what the prognosis will be.

There are also times that I cry out, "Please don't leave now, we finally connected, nurturing and loving."

As the family gathers, I notice old, ingrained, familiar dynamics unfolding. Five days later, the doctors knew there was no possible recovery.

The damage was done.

I let her go softly, gently.

I hold her arm, stroke her hair, and help her breathe her last breath.

A few days later, I notice I'm dropping things for the first time in eight years. I know this isn't about my mother's death, but the tension and control that filled the air like black smoke.

That's when the words by Dr. Horowitz take on a new meaning:

You are all about epigenetics.

The healers saw only part of the story. His words gift me a new direction.

When I returned home four weeks after the funeral, I began my deep dive into the scientific field of epigenetics.

I learned that epigenetics is the study of how our environment, beliefs, behaviors, and experiences influence gene expression without altering the DNA code itself.

And I know, in that moment, that I'm opening another door and eager to walk through it.

I ask myself: *How will the role of epigenetics help me unravel the traumas I carry, not just from my own life, but the generations before me?*

As I delved into medical and scientific research, I reviewed my healing history and started connecting the dots.

My parents' beliefs and unhealed pain are living in my cells, encoded into my energetic and epigenetic system.

CHANGE THE EXPRESSION OF THE EXPERIENCE

What if I can change the expression of the traumatic experience? I can't change the actual event, but I can change how my body energetically and emotionally holds it!

Knowing I carried my parents' unhealed wounds, I grew curious about how those wounds show up in my physical and emotional body.

I became a researcher in my very own laboratory.

Do wounds show up as emotional triggers, chronic pain, maybe even disease? As depression, avoidance, addiction, and confusion?

I understand that to heal trauma truly, we must change the expression of the experience in our cells. I decide to put my research to work.

One day, while taking my morning walk, I stopped dead in my tracks. I am in the middle of the street. I'm overcome with feelings and desperate for change.

Laura, it's time to shift your first trauma—your birth trauma.

My mother told me in my early teens that my father chased her down nine flights of stairs with a gun when she was seven months pregnant with me. She went into labor two hours after the event. I was born two months prematurely.

It's time to put my money where my mouth is and use the healing tool I created. The tool is aptly named, *The CoreRestore Healing Method.*

I begin the process and allow the energy to guide me. I'm ready to role-play both my mother and father.

Role-playing my mother:

I'm running down the stairs away from my husband, who is chasing me with a gun. Suddenly, I stop, turn around, and look into his eyes.

I say calmly, "Stop. If you want to kill me, then kill me. If you don't, you are scaring our unborn baby."

My father stops. He sits down on the step and places his gun beside him. He then buries his face in his hands and begins to cry.

"I am terrified of dying."

I walk away. I feel the weight of what I carried for sixty-four years slip off my shoulders.

Shortly after returning home, I had a huge aha moment:

He was armed, and I became disarmed.

After the roleplay, I never again feared being chased by a man with a gun. I felt a profound sense of freedom. This powerful tool helped me release, resolve, and eradicate this inherited imprint that I carried from my parents' unhealed wounds.

I have used the CoreRestore process on every traumatic event I can recall in my life. This tool focuses on releasing inherited burdens and restoring your sense of inner wholeness.

Now it's your turn to try this process.

Open your heart to changing whatever you feel needs to be addressed. It can be a life-changing experience, as it has been for me.

My wish is that you gain a new perspective on what drives you and how you want to show up in the world. Your life—your actions, reactions, beliefs, and desires—can finally become yours, not your parents', not your grandparents', not their unhealed realities.

THE TOOL

The purpose of the CoreRestore Healing Method is to go to the core to heal so much more. We hold experiences from our lifetime and our parents' lifetimes deep within our cells. That's the place to visit.

It's the space we all embody—in between our busy minds and our natural flow of brilliant energy! This is where we change the expression of our epigenetics and live authentically.

- To begin, take a moment to recall a life event that you experienced, or you've been told has affected you.

- Sit with the experience and feel your body's response.

- Notice your sensibilities.

- Remember, you always want to be in a place where you feel energetically connected to a quiet, peaceful, safe space. This can be in your home, your garden, the woods, beach—anywhere you feel fully present in your body.

Note: If you enter this space with curiosity and open-hearted desire for transformation and resolution, it will support you in the role-play, and you'll feel more grounded. If at any time this feels overwhelming, stop. Please appreciate what you were able to do and give yourself a hug for having the willingness to explore.

Next:

- Decide on a particular life event you'd like to role-play. Choose a memory that has lingered for years. The process will be clearer, so you feel more at ease; for example, a misunderstanding or a troubling experience.

- Begin by stepping into the intuitive energy field—what I refer to as the knowing field—welcoming only pure energy. This is the place that feels safe and peaceful.

- Drop into the energy of your body, which naturally quiets the mind. In this softened space, unhealed trauma often rises to the surface.

- Step into the role of the parent (or person) you want to change to express the experience.

- Speak to them in a tone of resolution and understanding. Stay centered and aligned.

- Feel into the opening as you change the expression.

- Breathe and release.

How do you feel? Did you experience an AHA moment of release and renewal?

Can you sense an energetic and emotional shift? Write down or voice record your release. Did this tool help you release an inherited energetic imprint you've been carrying from your parents?

If you enjoyed this healing tool and have questions, visit my website and send me a message.

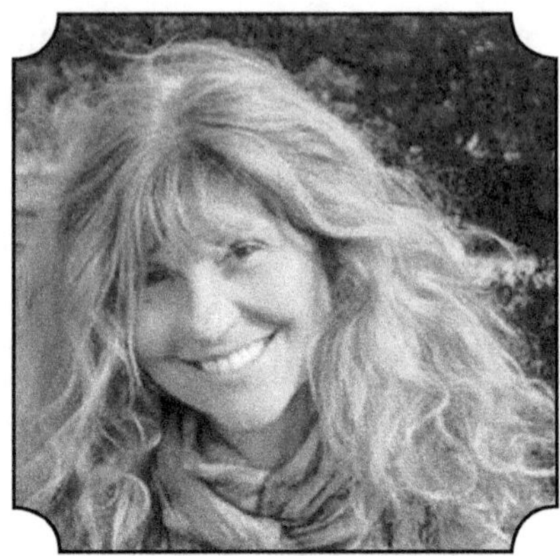

Laura Mayer, M.A., OTR, founder of *Opening Doorways Healing Practice,* bridges her clinical expertise with intuitive knowing. With over three decades of experience as a licensed occupational therapist in adult psychiatry and pediatrics, her work reflects a rare fusion of science and soul. She is an epigenetic healer, author, OT consultant, and Paint-Intuit.

Laura's profound healing journey led her deep into the realms of intuition and mysticism, where she explored alternative modalities and embodied wisdom. She now helps others open the doors to transformation by flawlessly weaving medical training with healing intuition, creative expression, and spiritual guidance.

Her specialty now lies in epigenetic healing—supporting individuals in releasing inherited emotional wounds and energetic imprints that no longer serve them. Laura's soul purpose is in offering her clients a holographic healing experience, where she receives guidance directly from Source and translates the information with a mystical depth and compassionate presence for integration and resolution.

As the creator of The CoreRestore Healing Method and HeART Energetic Expression, she bridges truth, healing, and creative expression through her transformational process. While her work is primarily focused on individual sessions, she also offers HeART Energetic Expression workshops for those seeking to unlock their deepest healing potential through the language of art, energy, and heart-centered presence.

Laura is the author of *Unlocking the Invisible Child* and a contributing co-author of the bestselling *Adventures in Manifesting and Healing from Within* series. Her upcoming second book, *Why Do I Feel This Way?*, continues to share her golden thread of transformation and truth.

When she's not in Europe, Laura is hanging with her puppy Jules or painting the next intuitive hit that comes through. She loves walking, dancing, and engaging in deep esoteric conversation.

Connect with Laura:

Website: https://www.laurajmayer.com

Instagram: https://www.instagram.com/paint_intuit

Facebook: https://www.facebook.com/laura.mayer.52035

Email: laura@laurajmayer.com

Allow with an Open Heart:

To accept divine light and energy.

To continue to meet in the all.

To travel the galaxy amongst the stars.

Shining the light of unconditional
love in all its forms.

~ R. Scott Holmes

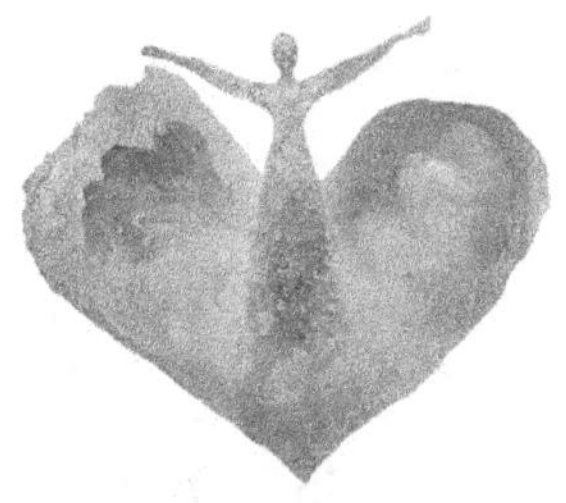

CHAPTER 25

ALLOWING THE WAY
CREATE YOUR DREAM LIFE THROUGH PRESENCE

R. Scott Holmes

Allow, with Ease

> The wisdom of your guides.
>
> To hear the wisdom of intention.
>
> To accept the journey as it unfolds.
>
> Revealing the mountains, the valleys, the deserts, and the shores.

Allow, with Grace

> Each encounter wrapped in compassion.
>
> Each judgement as it slides away.
>
> Each connection to grow as it will.
>
> Creating a world of grounded peace, love, and understanding.

Allow, with an Open Heart

To accept divine light and energy.

To continue to meet in the all.

To travel the galaxy amongst the stars.

Shining the light of unconditional love in all its forms.

MY STORY

I've been writing and diving so deep, trying to tell my story this past month.

How can I possibly share the tidal wave of emotions when I lost my wife?

How do I express the sheer devastation of losing my daughter?

How can I describe the depth of despair I experienced when words seem so empty and hollow?

Hemali Vora invited me to write in the collaboration *Sacred Death* for Brave Healer Productions. I had no idea how profound my "yes" would resonate.

It changed my life.

I have written in thirteen collaborations. I'm involved in three podcasts a month, interviewing men and women from around the world. I've traveled to three continents, seventeen countries, and so much of the United States. I get to write, coach, speak, and teach. It all started with a simple "yes" to the hardest thing I've ever done—allow.

It was a long road for thirty years with my wife, Moira's journey through breast cancer. After losing our youngest daughter, we continued living as best we could through the sorrow always bubbling close to the surface. Moira's last few years were filled with hospital visits, longer and longer hospital stays, and finally, the last few months at home.

I was lost, my world shrunk to rambling around the empty house, when my friend Paul called and we went to lunch.

I strained to hear Paul in the noisy café as we reminisced about our plans to travel after college. I settled down and had a family while Paul traveled the globe, started multiple businesses, and then found that life with children was what he needed.

"Why don't we recreate the adventure we always talked about? Europe, but not as poor students." We were both just turning sixty.

I was unencumbered with caregiving for the first time in 35 years, and the chance to finally see Europe after all these years called to me.

Am I selfish in taking this trip? Could I? Should I?

Disembarking from the Iberia Airlines jet in Munich had me pinching myself. The 17-day driving journey was about to start. We settled into a black Audi Q7 diesel SUV for the ride of our lives: 2500 miles and infinite memories.

We traveled through Munich, Nuremberg, Furth, Dresden, and Mannheim, Germany; Prague, Czech Republic; Strasbourg, France; Basel, Geneva, Lausanne, Lucerne, and Zurich, Switzerland; Lake Cuomo and Venice, Italy; Ljubljana, Slovenia; Bratislava, Slovakia; Vienna, Linz, and Salzburg, Austria. We returned to Munich in time for Oktoberfest.

"Hey Paul, tomorrow is my 60th birthday. Let's do something extra special."

Paul planned the epic day—breakfast in Germany, lunch in France, dinner in Switzerland.

Here I am, celebrating with my friend in Europe. I never believed this was possible, yet here I am. I'm so glad I didn't allow my misgivings to take over. I finally allowed myself the treasure of knowing my worth.

For the first time in my life, I felt like I could allow life in as it came to me.

A teacher of mine suggested I investigate this publishing house, which was collaborating with writers focused on different modalities. I contacted Laura Di Franco, and she suggested I become an advanced reader for a compilation that was coming out. I could review the book before publication.

I'm just starting my energy journey and don't know my ass from a hole in the ground. How could anything I have to say be of value to anyone?

Laura emailed me and asked if she could put the review on the back cover of the book.

Are you kidding me? My eighteen-year-old self was ecstatic. *That is the most exciting thing in my very short wannabe-writing career.*

Trying to sound as professional as possible, I told her, "If you would like to use the quote, I don't mind." *Wow, my words are being seen!*

Two weeks later, Laura called and asked me to speak with a lead author about a book she was putting together. I contacted Hemali Vora, and we talked about grief, loss, and what they mean. I was honored to be asked to contribute, but how can I write 3,000 words about my story? I could barely share it with another living soul without breaking down.

Moira, the lifelong teacher, would ask me to share her story so others can learn and find comfort in those words. I'll do this to honor her.

It took me thirty sleepless days and nights to put my story into words. The right words. Grappling with all the emotions exhumed the loss of my daughter and wife. Tear-stained legal pads were the vehicle that transported my grief, happiness, sadness, and joy into being.

Is it good enough? What will my family say? Will anyone read this or even care about it?

Three revisions and numerous "Can you read this and tell me what you think?" requests later, with fear bursting at the seams, "Your Path is Revealed: Transforming from Caregiving to Self-Caring" in *Sacred Death: 25 Tools for Caregivers* was born. It's an Amazon bestseller for Brave Healer Productions.

This was a turning point in my life after dealing with the losses of my 15-year-old daughter, my 60-year-old wife, my lifelong identity, and the heaviness of grief that permeated every pore, every cell, every day.

I allowed my eighteen-year-old writer to come out. When I graduated from high school, all I wanted to do was write and teach. College started, and then life changed my direction and calling.

Sometimes, allowing takes on a whole other level of trust. I worked with Samantha a dozen times in many venues, and then this happened:

Indian meditation music played in the small office where Samantha, the medium, worked. Small statues, incense wafting throughout the tight space, brightly colored wall hangings, and cozy pillows made the space warm and welcoming.

"It's good seeing you again. Please sit, and we'll start the reading."

I don't know what I'm expecting. After these last few years, I need some direction—if I even have a direction.

As the reading started, Sam looked to her right and started having a conversation with someone I couldn't see.

"No, I don't understand. What is Penang? Tell him what? He must what? Wait, I don't understand!"

I sat in rapt attention. *What just happened?*

"The gentleman is one of your guides—older, long white beard, and very short on explanation. He said you're to go to the Burmese Hindu Temple in Penang to collect your soul parts. And I'm not sure what any of that means."

Well, if she didn't understand that, how the hell am I supposed to make sense of it?

We looked up Penang, an island off the coast of Malaysia. We looked up the Dhammikarama Burmese Temple, and sure enough, there was only one, with a 40-foot-tall, golden-robed Buddha. Collecting soul parts was something she'd heard about from a shaman, but she wasn't sure what the practice involved.

"What am I supposed to do about this?" I asked.

"This is about you and your guides; I'm just the messenger."

Paul and I were heading on a 17-day guided tour of Thailand, Cambodia, and Vietnam the next month. *How am I supposed to get to Malaysia?*

The experiences in Bangkok, Phnom Penh, Ho Chi Min City, Hoi An, Hanoi, and Ha Long Bay were otherworldly. There were times when, even though I'd never been to Southeast Asia, I felt at home. I couldn't shake the feeling that I had come here before.

One month after getting back from our whirlwind trip, I received an email from the tour company we used. A tour of Singapore and Malaysia was on the list. I opened the email and looked through the itinerary. Sure enough, the last destination was Penang, and the hotel was three blocks from the Burmese Temple.

How will I pull this off? Do I really want to travel halfway around the world on the word of someone I can't see and a medium who has no clue what to do?

"How would you like to take a trip that will take 24 hours on a plane?" I asked. "You won't know the language, may not like the food, you'll be on a bus with 30 other people, and it's going to be hot."

Patti paused for five seconds and said, "Sure, I'll go anywhere in the world with you."

Shaun, our tour guide in Malaysia, was five feet of energy, knowledge, and good humor. I explained why we were on the tour and that on the last day, I'd make a pilgrimage to the Burmese Temple in our free time.

The tour was stunning, showing the best of Malay culture, historic sites, and history. On the last day of the tour, Shaun announced, "We have an extra special stop. This is the Dhammikarama Burmese Temple, where you'll see the reclining Buddha and the majestic, 40-foot standing Buddha." He winked to let me know it was his gift to me.

The spotless marble floor in the open-air temple felt cool as I slowly walked toward the statue. Stunning in gold robes, the marble statue seemed to glow. Gold filigree symbols painted the walls.

What am I supposed to do now? I traveled thousands of miles to be here, and I don't understand any of this. If I just listen and feel into it, something will come to me.

Slowly, I opened myself up to possibility. "Those lost soul parts—if they're meant for me, I invite them to come home." In my mind's eye, three orbs of light descended from behind the Buddha and glided down through my crown chakra.

I heard, "Welcome home," and my heart felt like it would burst. I stood, transfixed, until a tap on my shoulder brought me back.

"We have to go; the bus is waiting." Slowly, I walked back with Patti arm-in-arm; we were the last ones on the bus.

It took me about a month after getting back to take in everything that happened on this once-in-a-lifetime trip. I allowed all the sights, sounds, connections, and experiences to fully find their place in my being. It transformed my understanding of who I was and what I could do.

The decision to go to Peru at the end of August through the beginning of September was difficult. I'd miss family functions and the beginning of the public school year, where I worked.

Going to Peru wasn't even on my top ten list. However, my internal guides instructed me to go—as it'd be the next step on my spiritual journey.

Over the last five years, my ever-present guardians pointed me to Thailand, Cambodia, Vietnam, Singapore, Malaysia, and India.

Each step was an important part of my understanding of the world and, more importantly, the journey to myself.

"You have to see the mountains on the side of the plane!"

This may be the most beautiful sunrise I've ever seen, even more beautiful than the beach succumbing to the early sun on Amelia Island.

I leaned awkwardly so my seat-mate could view the sun, casting light and dark shadows on the peaks.

The seventeen-hour trip to Cusco, Peru, in the middle of the Andes, concluded with the sun rising in front of the propellered, forty-seat plane looking over the sea of clouds with peaks of the mountains rising as islands in the sky, highlighted by sun and shadow.

Observing the grandeur Mother Earth provides from this vantage point allowed my excitement and anticipation to grow even stronger despite the travel weariness.

Little did I know how life-changing the next two weeks would be.

When we landed, twenty strangers from all walks of life, ages thirty to seventy-two, from across the US and Canada gathered.

Only knowing two of this traveling band previously allowed me to observe and settle in. In the midst of travel chaos and crowd noise, I breathed quietly.

The excitement of travel, where your senses are on high alert to take in every sight, sound, smell, and taste, kept my weariness at bay. Meeting each of these like-guided people was an opportunity to explore the connection.

Along with being guided through the heart of Peru by Jorge Luis Delgado, I had the opportunity to participate in Incan rituals and learn about (and understand) these ancient ceremonies celebrating Father Sun and Mother Earth. Warmth spreads through my heart as I realize: *This is only the beginning of my adventure.*

"It's only a moderate climb, so bring your hiking boots and poles if you need them."

Only two miles (and two and a half hours later), seemingly climbing straight up at times, we reached the top of a tiered temple, layered with structures, overlooking valleys on both sides.

Each of our band walked, trekked, and limped at times at their own pace, with helping hands extended as was needed to climb the uneven and sometimes perilous path ever upward.

I frequently stopped to catch my breath, only to lose it again as I viewed the incredible landscapes unfolding around each turn. Tiers of stone walls, several half a mile across, cascaded down the mountains.

How did they construct these structures? At this elevation and with incredible precision lasting thousands of years?

The joy I felt as I took my final step at the summit is indescribable.

What an accomplishment!

What a relief as the bus came into sight after our five-hour sojourn.

To the ancestors, this was only a stroll through the Andes.

It sounds trite, but the Universe keeps giving lessons until they are learned. We repeat the same patterns over and over. The lessons not learned—divorce, break-ups, bad jobs, family chaos—all are changed only when we change our perspective by being present.

What does that look like? Only you know that answer, as it's at the heart of what you're willing to allow.

My wild, untamed truth is that everything I thought, was taught, was trained in, and was conditioned into me shrank my world. I used to think I could control everything in my world because it was so small.

Spring forward to the present—I realize none of the boundaries, the fences, and the signposts are real. The rules are made up. I've travelled to the far side of the galaxy on magic carpet rides of unbelievability.

THE TOOL

The start of each one-on-one session is about allowing:

Get comfortable by sitting or lying down, comfortable and supported. Two deep inhales and exhales.

Allow the healing light and energy into your body. Allow it to flow where it needs to go. Just observe, don't force, no judgment. Just feel, observe, allow. This will be the hardest thing you will do today:

To allow whatever comes through to be seen and acknowledged.

To allow your darkest parts to come forward.

To allow the brilliance of healing light and unconditional love into your energetic body.

To allow yourself to listen to your body's inner wisdom.

To allow yourself to feel, observe, and be vulnerable through sound, image, physical sensations, or knowing.

Getting energetically cleared slows down the roller coaster your mind seems to be on. Grounding yourself to Mother Earth gives you the strength to stand tall and the stability to move forward. Aligning your energetic body creates lifelines of stamina and the ability to be present in every aspect of your life.

If you had clarity, strength, and stability in mind, body, and spirit, how might you show up differently in this world and for yourself?

From this starting point, clients have let loose the bonds of heavy energy carried for years, as this weight kept them tied down. Allowing breath into places long forgotten, every organ begins to work in alignment, smothered no more by the heavy chains that bound them.

How open do you have to be to see those parts of you? Are you ready to allow something you've carried your whole life to be cleared, never to return? Never to return to overwhelm your senses, thoughts, emotions, or your sense of self?

It's as simple and as hard as allowing the old stories to fade away and to start writing your present-day story.

Joy arises when we return to ourselves; when we ground our essence in the body, clear the energetic clutter, and release what no longer serves us. It's the quiet radiance that emerges when presence takes the lead and the soul feels safe enough to exhale.

In this space, joy becomes more than a feeling. It becomes a way of being.

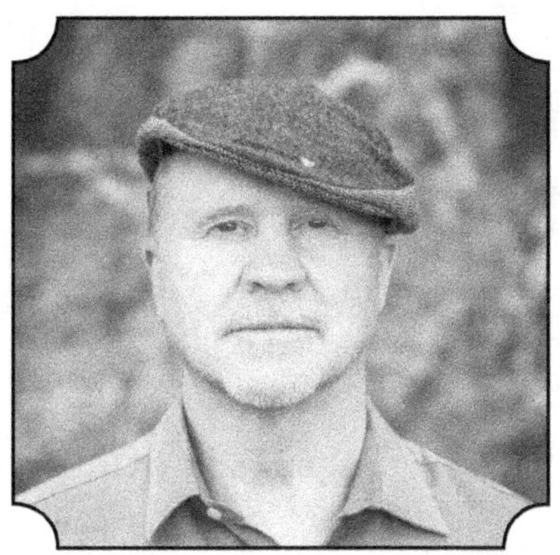

R. Scott Holmes is a quantum healing practitioner, transformational coach, and Amazon bestselling author whose work bridges science, spirit, and the human heart. A Reiki Master Teacher, Polarity Therapist, RYSE Teacher, Theta Healer, Universal White Time Healing Practitioner, and certified Find Your Voice Coach. Scott blends a decade of study with the hard-earned wisdom of lived experience.

Scott's path into holistic healing began in the depths of loss. After a 20-year caregiving journey with his wife and multiply-impaired daughter—and the passing of his wife of 39 years—he was guided into the world of energy, awareness, and transformation. Through this awakening, he discovered not only how to heal but also how to help others find meaning, freedom, and joy in their own lives.

Through one-on-one sessions, teaching, hospice volunteering, and his monthly podcasts, Scott has held sacred space for countless professionals and seekers, helping them remember who they are and reconnect to their innate wholeness. His collaborations with Brave Healer Productions capture the essence of his journey—honest, heart-centered explorations of resilience, authenticity, and the alchemy of healing.

When not teaching or writing, Scott can be found traveling the world with his wife, Patti—exploring sacred sites, tasting local cuisines, climbing mountains, and meditating by the sea. Yoga, Qigong, and daily meditation keep him grounded in gratitude, curiosity, and wonder for this extraordinary life we get to live.

Contact Scott for a free thirty-minute share to see if you can unwrap the questions carried in your heart.

Connect with Scott:

Website: https://rscottholmes.com/

Email: scott@rscottholmes.com

Facebook: https://www.facebook.com/scott.holmes.31105674

Instagram: https://www.instagram.com/r.scottholmes/

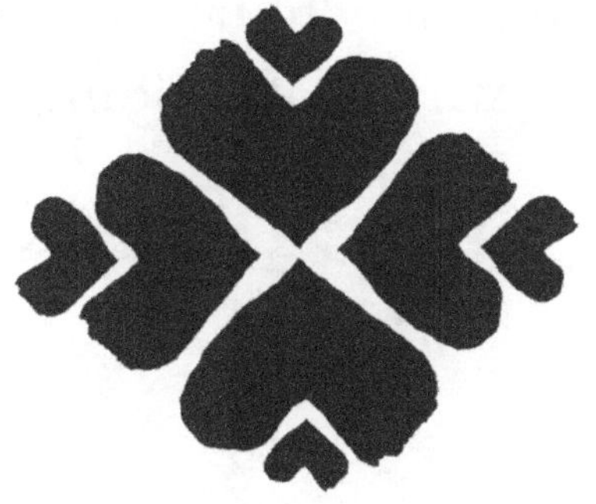

Trailblazing a new story
isn't always going to be liked by everyone.
That's what makes doing it brave.

~Laura Di Franco

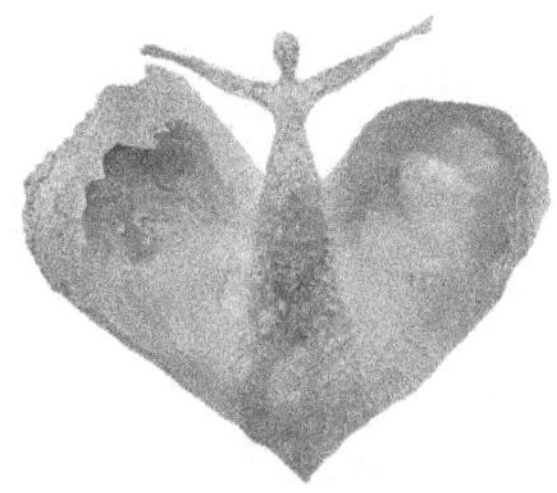

The Beginning of Your Journey Starts Today!

Dear Reader,

This is my love letter to you—a message from my heart to yours to help you realize our why and mission for this book. And this is way more than a book. It's a generous community of experts waiting for you to reach out.

You're not alone; if you don't have the solution yet, there's hope.

What if there's something you haven't learned yet that could change everything?

What else is possible when it comes to healing and living a better life?

This book has the solutions and answers to those questions, as well as a kind and powerful community willing to guide you.

Sometimes the most courageous thing you can do is reach out and ask that first question. These authors are waiting to assist and support you.

We hope you feel curious about the different modalities presented here and give the tools a try. Each author provides contact information so you can continue the conversation, ask your questions, and get help with the next steps on your journey. Take advantage of that opportunity!

You living your best, healthiest, most purposeful life is a gift to the world. You matter. Taking care of yourself is how you honor the body-mind-soul you are. When you ensure your own peak health, you make it possible to serve others. When you give yourself the gift of self-love and self-care, your light shines brighter and sparks joy in others.

Make yourself a priority. That is world-changing.

Every answer is within—and the tools in this book will help you connect with that inner healer and power.

With warrior love,

Laura

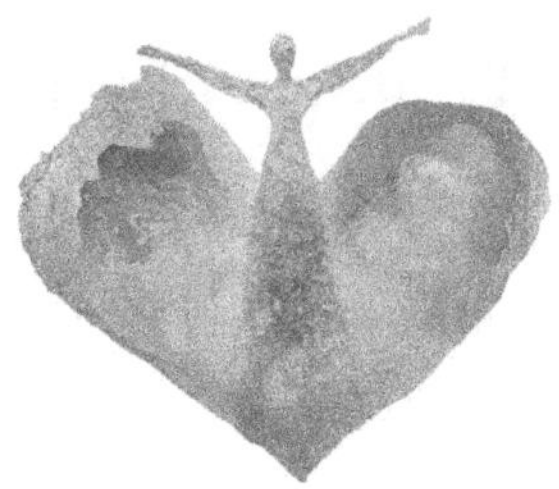

A Rampage of Gratitude

So many people make a book like this possible, and I'm so grateful for this village:

Our expert co-authors: You're the reason I get up every day with fire in my soul. Your passion, energy, enthusiasm, and love of writing are palpable, and I'm so grateful to you all for coming to the table in the spirit of collaboration. You're truly showing the world what's possible when a community comes together to change the world. Thank you.

Kelly vdH - Kaschula, our Brave Healer Productions Publishing Manager and Brave Kids Books Director, is also the interior designer for this book! Thank you for being my partner in everything that is Brave Healer Publishing and for sticking with me on the easy days and the stressful ones. Your friendship means everything to me. Thank you for your brilliant illustrations and interior design for this book.

Maggie McLaughlin, our Amazon and publishing pro: Thank you for being part of the team that gets every book to bestseller. Working with you makes every project a breeze. You're so good at what you do. The way you care about our projects makes them even more special.

Davide DeAngelis, our cover designer: This is a magnificent work of art that makes me proud to publish. I'm incredibly grateful for your artistic talent and ability to bring a cover vision to life.

The Brave Healer Book Launch Team, and every soul who has signed up to be an advanced reader for any of our books, thank you so much. You are the fuel for all of us here. Our purpose is you! Thank you.

All our readers (YOU!)—the amazing people who picked up our books and dove in to explore, learn, and grow—you're amazing, and we love you. You're never alone. We're so grateful for you, for your interest in our books, and for being brave enough to read and go on your own journey of healing.

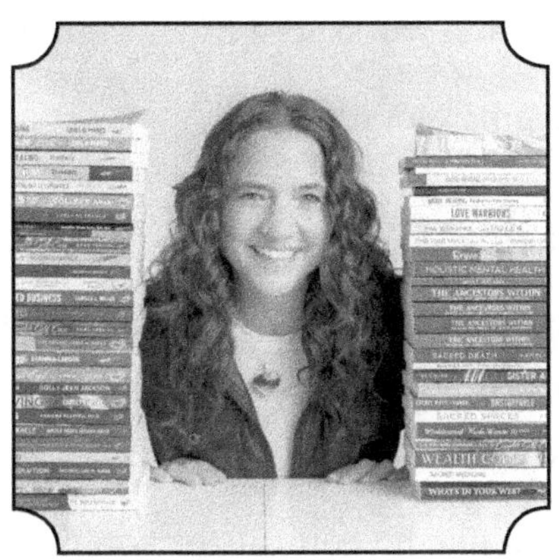

About the Lead Author

Laura Di Franco is the CEO of Brave Healer Productions (including Brave Business Books and Brave Kids Books), a multi-time award-winning publisher for holistic health, wellness, and business professionals who want to become bestselling authors, build their community and business, and leave their legacy in a more conscious way.

Laura holds a master's degree, has 30 years of experience in holistic physical therapy, is a third-degree black belt in Taekwondo, and is the author of 15 books. Brave Healer Productions has published over 100 Amazon bestselling books with a mission to help the world experience what's possible, one brave word at a time.

Laura is a divorced mom with two adult kids and one Jack Russell, a lover of the sunrise and dark chocolate, a spoken-word poet, an inspirational speaker, and is convinced she was a race car driver in a past life. She has a contagious passion for helping you share brave words that build your business and leave your legacy. Laura has a secret alien passion for big birds—eagles, hawks, owls, and other large feathered, flying objects regularly tell her, "You're on the right track; keep going!"

Want some advice about your book idea? Schedule a chat with our publishing team by reaching out to support@LauraDiFranco.com

Get access to The Brave Healer Resources Vault with thousands of hours of training, master classes, and workshops for author-entrepreneurs:

https://lauradifranco.com/resources-vault/

CONNECT WITH LAURA:

Website: https://BraveHealer.com

The Good Morning Joy Episode:
https://youtu.be/vvYyMJGpP_U?si=zstrMPEFxrB5wDxq

LinkedIn: https://www.linkedin.com/in/thelauradifranco/

YouTube:
https://www.youtube.com/c/BraveHealerProductionswithLauraDiFranco

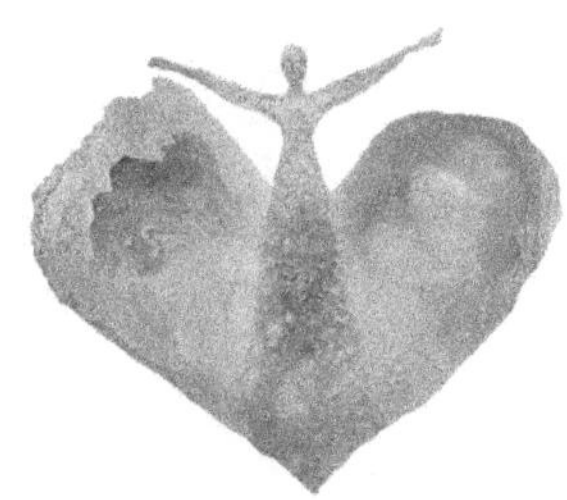

Books From Brave Healer Productions

Our company has published powerful expert collaborations and solo-authored books on many important topics, such as:

Abundance	Finding your voice	Motherhood
Abuse prevention	Grief	Networking
Ancestral healing	Healthy living	Poetry
Aging	Holistic healing	Purpose
Bravery	Human design	Rites and rituals
Breathwork	Intuition	Self-care
Business growth	Kindness	Self-healing
Caregiving	Leadership	Shamanic healing
Death	Legacy	Success
Empowerment	Love	Transformation
Energy medicine	Mental health	Writing
Entrepreneurship	Mentorship	
Expressive arts	Mindset	

Visit BraveHealer.com and the BOOKS tab to browse all our titles, including our children's books!

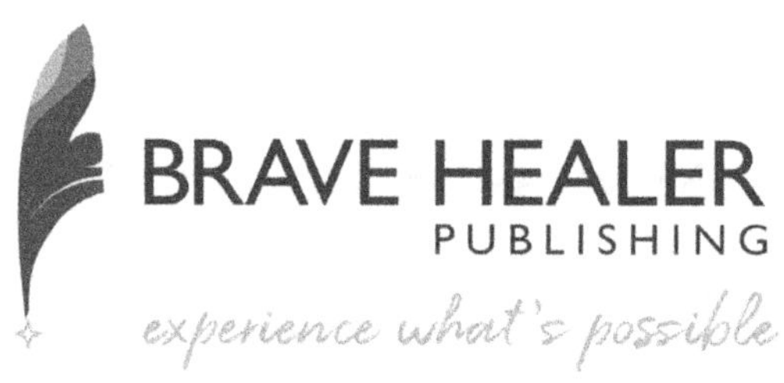

You were born, so you're worthy.

Your message matters.

What if the thing you're still a little afraid to
share is exactly the thing someone needs to hear
to change (or even save) their life?

It's time to be brave!